Oxford Case Histories in Lung Cancer

Oxford Case Histories

Series Editors

Sarah Pendlebury and Peter Rothwell

Published:

Neurological Case Histories (Sarah T. Pendlebury, Philip Anslow, and Peter M. Rothwell)

Oxford Case Histories in Anaesthesia (Jon McCormack and Keith Kelly)

Oxford Case Histories in Cardiology (Rajkumar Rajendram, Javed Ehtisham, and Colin Forfar)

Oxford Case Histories in Gastroenterology and Hepatology (Alissa J. Walsh, Otto C. Buchel, Jane Collier, and Simon P.L. Travis)

Oxford Case Histories in General Surgery (Judith Ritchie and K. Raj Prasad)

Oxford Case Histories in Geriatric Medicine (Sanja Thompson, Nicola Lovett, John Grimley Evans, and Sarah Pendlebury)

Oxford Case Histories in Respiratory Medicine (John Stradling, Andrew Stanton, Najib M. Rahman, Annabel H. Nickol, and Helen E. Davies)

Oxford Case Histories in Rheumatology (Joel David, Anne Miller, Anushka Soni, and Lyn Williamson)

Oxford Case Histories in TIA and Stroke (Sarah T. Pendlebury, Ursula G. Schulz, Aneil Malhotra, and Peter M. Rothwell)

Oxford Case Histories in Neurosurgery (Harutomo Hasegawa, Matthew Crocker, and Pawan Singh Minhas)

Oxford Case Histories in Oncology (Harutomo Hasegawa, Matthew Crocker, and Pawan Singh Minhas)

Oxford Case Histories in Sleep Medicine (Himender Makker, Matthew Walker, Hugh Selsick, Bhik Kotecha, and Ama Johal)

Oxford Case Histories in Lung Cancer

Himender Makker
Consultant Respiratory Physician, North Middlesex University
Hospital NHS Trust, London, UK

Adam Ainley
Specialist Registrar in Respiratory Medicine, National Heart and Lung
Institute, Imperial College, London, UK

Sanjay Popat
Consultant Thoracic Medical Oncologist, The Royal Marsden NHS
Foundation Trust, London, UK

Julian Singer
Consultant Clinical Oncologist, Princess Alexandra Hospitals NHS
Trust, Harlow, UK

Martin Hayward
Consultant Thoracic Surgeon and Clinical Lead for Thoracic
Surgery, University College London Hospitals NHS Foundation Trust,
London, UK

Antke Hagena
Consultant in Palliative Medicine, North Middlesex University
Hospital NHS Trust, London, UK

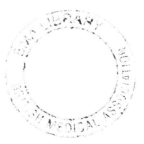

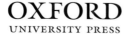

OXFORD
UNIVERSITY PRESS

OXFORD
UNIVERSITY PRESS

Great Clarendon Street, Oxford, OX2 6DP,
United Kingdom

Oxford University Press is a department of the University of Oxford.
It furthers the University's objective of excellence in research, scholarship,
and education by publishing worldwide. Oxford is a registered trade mark of
Oxford University Press in the UK and in certain other countries

Published in the United States of America by Oxford University Press
198 Madison Avenue, New York, NY 10016, United States of America

British Library Cataloguing in Publication Data

Data available

Library of Congress Control Number: 2018941862

ISBN 978–0–19–881303–3

Printed in Great Britain by
Ashford Colour Press Ltd, Gosport, Hampshire

Preface

There have been immense changes in the management of lung cancer over the last 20 years—from multidisciplinary models of care to innovations in diagnosis, staging, and treatment. We have better tools for quick and accurate diagnosis and staging, a rapidly expanding array of molecular and biological agents for treatment, novel approaches to deliver radiotherapy, and less invasive thoracic surgical techniques to treat lung cancer. We are beginning to see a distinct impact of these changes on lung cancer outcomes. We are likely to have more opportunities for cure with the introduction of screening for lung cancer.

This book reflects the current multidisciplinary approach to the management of lung cancer incorporating these changes. The layout of the book and sequence of case histories track the patient journey from presentation to diagnosis, staging, treatment options, and palliative care. Case histories in each section have been selected and written by experienced clinicians. Each case history provides a brief summary with relevant images followed by question and answers—commonly raised at multidisciplinary meetings.

It has been my greatest pleasure and privilege to work with my lung multidisciplinary team colleagues over the last 20 years to provide a lung cancer service, and I now have opportunity to share our experience with you in the form of this book. I am extremely grateful to my coauthor and contributor colleagues for taking time out from their busy schedules to contribute to the book.

Finally, I wish to offer my sincere thanks to Caroline Smith and her colleagues April Peake and Sylvia Warren at Oxford University Press for their constant support and help throughout this project.

Himender Makker

Contents

List of Abbreviations

AAH	atypical adenomatous hyperplasia		DNACPR	do not attempt cardiopulmonary resuscitation
ADRT	advance decision to refuse treatment		EBUS	endobronchial ultrasound
AED	antiepileptic drug		ECG	electrocardiogram
AF	atrial fibrillation		ECOG	Eastern Cooperative Oncology Group
AIS	adenocarcinoma in situ		EGFR	epidermal growth factor receptor
ALK	anaplastic lymphoma kinase			
ALT	alanine aminotransferase		EMA	European Medicines Agency
ASCO	American Society of Clinical Oncology		EML4	echinoderm microtubule-associated protein-like-4
AST	aspartate aminotransferase		EMN	electromagnetic navigation
AUC	area under the curve		EORTC	European Organisation for Research and Treatment of Cancer
AVP	arginine vasopressin			
BAC	bronchoalveolar carcinoma		ER	oestrogen receptor
BRAF	v-RAF murine sarcoma viral oncogene homologue B / B-Raf proto-oncogene serine/threonine kinase		ESMO	European Society of Medical Oncology
			EUS	endoscopic ultrasound
BTS	British Thoracic Society		FB	flexible bronchoscopy
CAV	cyclophosphamide, doxorubicin, and vincristine		FDA	US Food and Drug Administration
CEA	carcinoembryonic antigen		FDG	fludeoxyglucose
CI	confidence interval		FEV_1	forced expiratory volume for 1 second
CK	cytokeratin			
CNS	central nervous system		FLAIR	fluid-attenuated inversion recovery
COAD	chronic obstructive airway disease		FNA	fine needle aspiration
COPD	chronic obstructive pulmonary disease		FVC	forced vital capacity
			G-CSF	granulocyte–colony stimulating factor
COX	cyclo-oxygenase			
CPET	cardiopulmonary exercise test		GCT	granular cell tumour
CRP	C-reactive protein		GOLD	Global Initiative for Chronic Obstructive Lung Disease
CT	computed tomography			
ctDNA	circulating tumour DNA		GP	general practitioner
CTV	clinical target volume		GTV	gross tumour volume
DLCO	diffusing capacity for CO		H&E	haematoxylin and eosin
DLL3	Delta-like protein 3		HER	human epidermal growth factor receptor

HER2	erb-b2 receptor tyrosine kinase 2
HPF	high-powered field
HR	hazard ratio
IASLC	International Association for the Study of Lung Cancer
Ig	immunoglobulin
IHC	immunohistochemistry
IMCA	independent mental capacity advisor
IMIG	International Mesothelioma Interest Group
INR	international normalized ratio
IPF	idiopathic pulmonary fibrosis
irAE	immune-related adverse event
ITV	internal target volume
KRAS	Kirsten rat sarcoma viral oncogene homologue
LDH	lactate dehydrogenase
MASCC	Multinational Association for Supportive Care in Cancer
MCA	Mental Capacity Act
MDT	multidisciplinary team
MIA	minimally invasive adenocarcinoma
MPM	malignant pleural mesothelioma
MRI	magnetic resonance imaging
mTOR	mechanistic target$_{max}$ of rapamycin kinase
NCEPOD	National Confidential Enquiry into Patient Outcomes and Death
NET	neuroendocrine tumour
NLST	National Lung Screening Trial
NSAID	non-steroidal anti-inflammatory drug
NSCLC	non-small-cell lung cancer
OR	odds ratio
ORR	objective response rate
PAP	pulmonary artery pressure
PCA	patient-controlled analgesia
PCI	prophylactic cranial irradiation

PD-1	programmed cell death-1
PD-L1	programmed death ligand-1
PET	positron emission tomography
PgR	progesterone receptor
PIK3CA	phosphatidylinositol-4,5-bisphosphate 3-kinase catalytic subunit alpha
PPI	proton pump inhibitor
ppoDLCO	predicted postoperative DLCO
ppoFEV$_1$	predicted postoperative FEV$_1$
PRN	pro re nata
PSA	prostate specific antigen
RCC	Anti-renal cell carcinoma antigen
R-EBUS	radial–endobronchial ultrasound
ROS-1	ROS proto-oncogene 1 receptor tyrosine kinase
ROSE	rapid on-site evaluation
RPA	recursive partitioning analysis
SABR	stereotactic ablative radiotherapy
S$_a$O$_2$	amount of oxygen bound to haemoglobin in arterial blood
SCC	squamous cell carcinoma
SCLC	small-cell lung cancer
SIADH	syndrome of inappropriate antidiuretic hormone
SRE	skeletal-related event
SUV	standardized uptake value
SVCO	superior vena cava obstruction
TBNA	transthoracic needle biopsy
TKI	tyrosine kinase inhibitor
TLCO	transfer factor of the lung for carbon monoxide
TNM	tumour–node–metastasis
TPDS	tumour predisposition syndrome
TTE	transthoracic echocardiogram
TTF-1	thyroid transcription factor-1
UICC	Union for International Cancer Control
US	ultrasound

VALG	Veterans Administration Lung Study Group
VATS	video-assisted thoracoscopic surgery
VCO_2	carbon dioxide production
VEGFR-2	vascular endothelial growth factor receptor-2
VO_2	respiratory oxygen uptake

VO_2max	maximum rate of oxygen consumption which remains unchanged during a staged increase in incremental exercise
VTE	venous thromboembolism
WBRT	whole brain radiation therapy
WHO	World Health Organization

Contributors

Adam Ainley
Specialist Registrar in Respiratory Medicine, National Heart and Lung Institute, Imperial College, London, UK

Spyros Gennatas
Clinical Research Fellow, National Heart and Lung Institute, Imperial College, London, UK

Rebecca Gillibrand
Consultant Cellular Pathologist, North Middlesex University Hospital NHS Trust, London, UK

Antke Hagena
Consultant in Palliative Medicine, North Middlesex University Hospital NHS Trust, London, UK

Martin Hayward
Consultant Thoracic Surgeon and Clinical Lead for Thoracic Surgery, University College London Hospitals NHS Foundation Trust, London, UK

Adam Januszewski
Academic Clinical Fellow, The Royal Marsden NHS Foundation Trust, London, UK

Oscar Juan
Medical Oncologist, University Hospital La Fe, Valencia, Spain

Sashin Kaneria
Consultant Radiologist, North Middlesex University Hospital NHS Trust, London, UK

Himender Makker
Consultant Respiratory Physician, North Middlesex University Hospital NHS Trust, London, UK

Sofoklis Mitsos
Cardiothoracic Surgery Clinical Fellow, University College London Hospitals NHS Foundation Trust, London, UK

Nikolaos Panagiotopoulos
Consultant Thoracic Surgeon, University College London Hospitals NHS Foundation Trust, London, UK

Davide Patrini
Senior Fellow in Cardiothoracic Surgery, University College London Hospitals NHS Foundation Trust, London, UK

Sanjay Popat
Consultant Thoracic Medical Oncologist, The Royal Marsden NHS Foundation Trust, London, UK

Bryan Sheinman
Consultant Chest Physician, North Middlesex University Hospital NHS Trust, London, UK

Julian Singer
Consultant Clinical Oncologist, Princess Alexandra Hospitals NHS Trust, Harlow, UK

Kobika Sritharan
Oncology Registrar, North Middlesex University Hospital NHS Trust, London, UK

Nadza Tokaca
Academic Clinical Fellow, The Royal Marsden NHS Foundation Trust, London, UK

Section I

Epidemiology, presentation, diagnosis, and staging

Case 1

Lung cancer in a 53 year old smoker

Adam Ainley, Rebecca Gillibrand, and Himender Makker

Case history

A 53 year old male was referred to the chest clinic because of persistent abnormalities seen on chest x-rays following an admission to hospital for treatment of left-sided community-acquired pneumonia. He had had an intermittent unproductive cough, breathlessness, and wheeze for 3 months that had been attributed to chronic obstructive pulmonary disease (COPD). He was a current smoker of 40 pack-years. On examination there was no abnormality. Chest x-rays demonstrated a persistent left lower zone abnormality and a chest CT scan revealed a left lower lobe mass with left hilar (9 mm) and paratracheal lymphadenopathy (15 mm). There were bilateral mid-zone pulmonary nodules and a small pleural effusion. PET-CT showed a fludeoxyglucose (FDG)-avid 3.3 × 3.2 cm left lower lobe mass with increased uptake, an 11 mm right lower lobe nodule, and subcarinal, pretracheal, and left hilar lymph node enlargement. No extrapulmonary lesions were noted. Fibreoptic bronchoscopy showed no endobronchial tumour; however, bronchial washings revealed several groups of atypical cells with a high nuclear–cytoplasmic ratio, nuclear hyperchromasia, and nuclear pleomorphism. The appearances, although not diagnostic, were suspicious for a non-small-cell carcinoma. CT-guided biopsy of the left lower lobe mass revealed cores of lung tissue infiltrated by tumour cells expressing cytokeratin 7 (CK7) and thyroid transcription factor-1 (TTF-1). CK20 and CK5/6 were negative. These features were consistent with a diagnosis of pulmonary malignancy.

Questions

1. What type of pulmonary malignancy are the patient's investigation results consistent with?

2. How do you differentiate primary adenocarcinoma of the lung from metastatic adenocarcinoma?

3. What further investigations should be considered in light of the tumour subtype diagnosed?

4. How would you stage this patient's disease?

5. How does the new TNM 8 classification differ from the TNM 7 staging system?

Answers

1. What type of pulmonary malignancy are the patient's investigation results consistent with?

The findings are consistent with a diagnosis of primary lung adenocarcinoma. This is the commonest subtype of lung cancer and accounts for approximately 50% of all lung cancers.

Lung cancer is one of the commonest cancer accounting for 20% of all cancers. There are four main subtypes: non-small-cell lung cancers (NSCLCs), including adenocarcinoma; squamous cell carcinoma and large-cell carcinoma; and small-cell lung cancer (SCLC). Eighty per cent of primary lung cancers are NSCLCs and 20% are SCLCs.

The diagnosis of lung cancer and subtyping requires cytology and/or a histological biopsy specimen. In most patients this is obtained by non-surgical methods such as fibreoptic bronchoscopy or under image (CT/US) guidance. Fibreoptic bronchoscopy is one of the commonest methods for obtaining cytological (bronchial washing and brushing) and/or biopsy (e.g. of an endobronchial tumour) specimens. However, the usefulness of conventional fibreoptic bronchoscopy has declined due to a change in the distribution pattern of lung cancer from central to peripheral disease. The introduction of endobronchial ultrasound (EBUS) bronchoscopy sampling of submucosal tumours and hilar and mediastinal lymph nodes has improved the diagnostic yield over that of conventional bronchoscopy.

CT-directed biopsy is required for the diagnosis of peripheral lung and pleural lesions. Sputum cytology, despite having a high specificity, is rarely used because of its low sensitivity.

The diagnosis of lung adenocarcinoma is based on the typical morphological features of glandular differentiation, including gland formation and mucin production. Different architectural patterns may be seen, including: lepidic (formerly bronchoalveolar); acinar; papillary; micropapillary; and solid. Cytologically, tumour cells typically have pleomorphic nuclei, prominent nucleoli, and vacuolated cytoplasm. However, poorly differentiated adenocarcinoma loses its characteristic architectural and morphological features and as such immunohistochemical staining is required.

Primary lung adenocarcinomas typically express CK7 and TTF-1. P63 and CK5/6 are usually negative—expression of these antibodies with negative expression of CK7 and TTF-1 would favour a squamous cell carcinoma.

2. How do you differentiate primary adenocarcinoma of the lung from metastatic adenocarcinoma?

The lung is a common site for secondary spread from tumours of the breast, colon, prostate, and kidney (renal cell carcinoma). Most pulmonary metastases are adenocarcinomas and it is important to establish if an adenocarcinoma is primary or metastatic in order to inform correct prognosis and treatment. The morphological features of primary and metastatic adenocarcinomas can be very similar and a panel of antibodies for immunohistochemical analysis is often useful.

CK7 and TTF-1 are expressed in the majority of lung adenocarcinomas (although 20% may be TTF-1 negative). Napsin A is also commonly expressed.

The other antibodies chosen should be selected depending on other possible primary sites. CK20 and CDX-2 are usually expressed by adenocarcinomas from the lower gastrointestinal tract. Oestrogen receptor (ER) and progesterone receptor (PgR) may be expressed by primary breast carcinomas; prostate-specific antigen (PSA) may be positive in metastatic prostate carcinoma; and Anti-renal cell carcinoma antigen (RCC) in renal carcinomas.

3. What further investigations should be considered in light of the tumour subtype diagnosed?

There have been tremendous advances in the treatment of advanced NSCLC with immunotherapy and targeted therapy. The effectiveness of these agents depends on the expression of certain types of tumour markers/mutations. Programmed cell death-1 (PD-1) protein suppresses killer cell T lymphocytes. Lung cancers expressing programmed death ligand-1 (PD-L1) deactivate T cells by binding to PD-1. Immunotherapy treatments targeted to either PD-1 or PD-L1 allow activated T cells to kill the tumour.

Epidermal growth factor receptor (EGFR) belongs to the family of receptor tyrosine kinases and plays an essential role in regulating cell proliferation, adhesion, and migration. Approximately 20–30% of lung adenocarcinomas have an EGFR mutation. Anaplastic lymphoma kinase (ALK) is another type of receptor tyrosine kinase and is expressed by 3–5% of primary lung adenocarcinomas. Patients with ALK or EGFR mutations may respond to targeted therapy using tyrosine kinase inhibitors (TKIs) and as such mutation analysis for these mutations should be considered for patients found to have an adenocarcinoma.

[Further discussion regarding the current recommendations for testing can be found in Case 11.]

4. How would you stage this patient's disease?

The tumour was reported to be 3.3 cm in diameter (T2) with evidence of hilar and mediastinal lymph node involvement (N2) and metastasis in the contralateral lung (M1a); thus, stage IV adenocarinoma of the lung (T2N2M1) on the basis of the TNM 7 staging classification.

TNM staging for lung cancer is based on tumour size, lymph node involvement, and metastasis.

Lung tumour size is assessed either on a surgically resected specimen (stages I, II, IIIA) or on PET-CT scan. It is recommended that tumour size is measured at the largest diameter. There is a good correlation between tumour size (T stage) measured on imaging (chest x-ray, PET-CT) and that measured on a surgically resected lung cancer except in patients with tumours associated with collapse/consolidation and surrounding oedema. CT may overestimate tumour size in these patients and PET-CT scan is likely to provide a more accurate tumour size. Accurate tumour localization and measurement on PET-CT scan helps not only with correct tumour staging but also with radiotherapy planning.

Nodal (hilar, mediastinal, and extrathoracic lymph node) staging is key to establishing surgically resectable/curable disease and avoiding futile thoracotomy. Nodal staging is based on the size of lymph nodes on CT scan: a lymph node of >1 cm on the short axis diameter is considered to be abnormal. However, the sensitivity (55%) and specificity (81%) of nodal spread based on the above CT criteria are poor. Although a PET-CT-positive node (increased uptake on PET scan) is a better predictor of nodal involvement (sensitivity 77%; specificity 86%), it is not sufficient to rule it out. EBUS is recommended for confirmation of nodal involvement in patients with enlarged nodes on CT scan or PET-positive lymph nodes. EBUS has a much better sensitivity (90%) and negative predictive value. In patients undergoing surgical resection for stage I and II lung cancer, mediastinal dissection and staging are recommended, even in the absence of lymph node involvement on CT or PET scan.

Staging of metastasis in most patients with histologically confirmed primary lung cancer is based on imaging. However, in patients with solitary or oligometastatic disease histological confirmation is usually required, particularly if the metastasis has an atypical appearance on CT scan or equivocal uptake on PET scan. Furthermore, the expression of tumour markers can differ between primary and metastatic disease, influencing the choice of biological agent—a significant proportion of patients with EGFR-negative primary lung cancer have EGFR-positive metastases.

5. How does the new TNM 8 classification differ from the TNM 7 staging system?

The TNM 7 classification was published in 2009 and implemented in 2010. Since then there have been major changes in the understanding of solitary pulmonary nodules as a result of low-dose CT screening trails. The most updated edition, the TNM 8 classification, was first published in 2017.

The new classification has proposed changes in T staging but has retained cut-offs of tumour size of 2 cm, 3 cm, 5 cm, and 7 cm; it has also introduced new cut-offs of 1 cm and 4 cm. The T1 cut-off remains at tumours of <3 cm but this has been subclassified into T1a <1 cm, T1b >1 cm to 2 cm, and T1c >2 cm to 3 cm. This has resulted in reclassification of stage I lung cancer into stage IA, IB and IC. Validation studies have confirmed the prognostic discriminatory value of this classification.

The T2 tumour size of >3 cm to 5 cm has been subclassified into T2a >3 cm to 4 cm and T2b >4 cm to 5 cm. There are no changes to the T3 and T4 classifications except that tumour invading the diaphragm is now staged as T4.

Stage III has been reclassified into stage IIIA, IIIB, and IIIC. Locally advanced lung cancer of T3 and T4 with N3 and M0 disease has been classified as IIIC. It has a similar prognosis to stage IVA disease but management approaches differ between stage IIIC and IVA lung cancer.

Stage IV lung cancer includes a wide range of disease from large intrathoracic tumours to multiple metastases. In patients with stage IV lung cancer the disease burden and management differ. A more accurate staging of stage IV disease has been recommended in the new TNM classification. Metastatic disease has been reclassified into M1a intrathoracic metastasis, M1b single extrathoracic metastasis, and M1c multiple metastatic disease. This restages stage IV cancers into stage IVA as intrathoracic disease and single-site extrathoracic metastasis and into stage IVB as multiple metastases.

Further reading

Goldstraw P et al. The IASLC Lung Cancer Staging Project: proposals for revision of the TNM stage groupings in the forthcoming (eighth) edition of the TNM Classification for Lung Cancer. J Thorac Oncol. 2016 Jan;11(1):39–51.

Rami-Porta R, Asamura H, Travis WD, Rusch VW. Lung cancer—major changes in the American Joint Committee on Cancer eighth edition cancer staging manual. CA Cancer J Clin. 2017 Mar;67(2):138–55.

Travis WD et al. Diagnosis of lung cancer in small biopsies and cytology: implications of the 2011 International Association for the Study of Lung Cancer/American Thoracic Society/European Respiratory Society classification. Arch Pathol Lab Med. 2013 May;137(5):668–84.

Case 2

Lung cancer in an ex-smoker with underlying lung fibrosis

Adam Ainley and Himender Makker

Case history

A 70 year old white female with a history of idiopathic pulmonary fibrosis (IPF) was referred to the respiratory clinic because of worsening breathlessness and a persistent dry cough. Her exercise tolerance had markedly worsened over the last year. She had lost weight over the last 4 months despite a normal appetite. Her past medical history included essential hypertension and hypercholesterolaemia. She was an ex-smoker, having stopped 10 years previously with a 15 pack-year history.

On examination she had bilateral basal crepitations and was hypoxic at rest with an S_aO_2 of 86% on room air. Her lung function tests were stable with a forced vital capacity (FVC) of 1.9 L (82% of predicted) and a forced expiratory volume for 1 second (FEV_1) of 1.70 L (86% of predicted) and gas transfer of 3.72 mmol/m/kPa (53% of predicted). Her chest x-ray was abnormal (Fig. 2.1) and a CT scan of her chest was requested on the basis of this (Fig. 2.2).

Questions

1. What are the notable abnormalities seen on the patient's chest x-ray and CT scan?
2. What are the known risk factors for lung malignancy?
3. How should patients with known risk factor(s) for lung cancer be monitored?

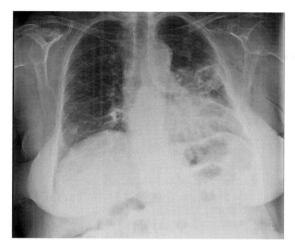

Fig. 2.1 Chest x-ray.

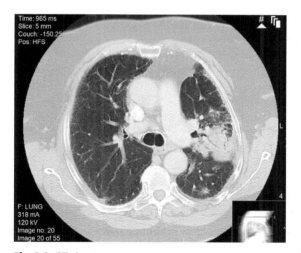

Fig. 2.2 CT chest.

Answers

1. What are the notable abnormalities seen on the patient's chest x-ray and CT scan?

The chest x-ray showed a left mid-zone opacification with a central translucent area, and CT confirmed a left mid-zone consolidation with an air bronchogram and a peripheral small area of opacity in addition to background changes of pulmonary fibrosis. Although these findings could be due to a superimposed pneumonia or worsening fibrosis, in an ex-smoker with IPF and a clinical picture of worsening shortness of breath and cough the possibility of lung cancer, and in particular bronchoalveolar carcinoma, should be considered.

Among the four main types of lung cancer adenocarcinoma is the most common (50%), followed by squamous cell, small-cell, and large-cell lung cancer. Over the last 50 years there has been a change in the prevalence of the different types of lung cancer with adenocarcinoma becoming more common, whereas the prevalence of squamous cell carcinoma has declined. Adenocarcinoma typically presents as a peripheral lung cancer while squamous cell carcinoma affects the central airways. This change in prevalence has been attributed to changes in smoking patterns—with a greater depth of inhalation required for the newer types of cigarettes than for older, non-tipped cigarettes—thus exposing more peripheral airways to carcinogens.

Bronchoalveolar carcinoma is a subtype of adenocarcinoma of the lung and accounts for approximately 6% of all lung cancers. It arises from epithelial cells located in terminal bronchioles and usually presents as peripheral disease. It typically grows along intact alveolar septum (lepidic growth pattern) and spreads into both the airways and lymphatic system. The radiographic features of bronchoalveolar carcinoma are quite variable compared with other types of lung cancer. The main radiological presentations of the lepidic type are as a solitary nodule of variable density (ground glass to solid), focal consolidation, and multifocal diffuse disease. The ground-glass opacity nodule is one of the most common presentations and is difficult to distinguish from inflammatory shadowing, a focal area of pulmonary fibrosis, or atypical adenomatous hyperplasia. A consolidative form is seen in about one-third of patients and tends to be of the mucinous histological type. It typically presents as a non-resolving pneumonia and, as such, the radiological finding of non-resolving peripheral consolidation pneumonia, especially associated with nodular changes, should raise the possibility of a bronchoalveolar carcinoma.

Case history continued

The patient's imaging and case were discussed at the lung cancer multidisciplinary team (MDT) meeting and it was decided that she should proceed to further investigations to obtain a histological diagnosis. She subsequently underwent a flexible bronchoscopy with biopsies taken that confirmed a diagnosis of bronchoalveolar carcinoma.

2. What are the known risk factors for lung malignancy?

Lung cancer occurs in 10–30% of patients with IPF. Most lung cancers associated with IPF are squamous cell carcinoma and are not located at the site of fibrosis but in separate peripheral areas.

Bronchoalveolar carcinoma is relatively rare in IPF. Although the radiological appearance of bronchoalveolar carcinoma can vary from nodular to diffuse changes, most patients with known pulmonary fibrosis present with ill-defined lesions mimicking air space consolidation. In patients with IPF it can be a cause of worsening breathlessness and dry cough.

Overall, tobacco (cigarette smoking) remains the most common and clearly identifiable risk factor for lung cancer. The relationship between tobacco smoking and the risk of lung cancer is well known. There is relatively little difference between the types of tobacco smoking—cigarette, cigar, or pipe smoking. Similarly there is relatively little difference in the risk of lung cancer with smoking different types of cigarettes, such as filtered cigarettes versus non-filtered cigarettes or low-tar and standard cigarettes. The main carcinogens in tobacco smoke are polycyclic aromatic carbons and tobacco-specific nitrosamines butane. The risk of lung cancer diminishes after tobacco cessation, but never returns to that of a life-long non-smoker. There is a negligible reduction in risk during the first 5 years of tobacco smoking cessation. Passive inhalation of tobacco smoke or environmental tobacco smoke is also a risk factor for lung cancer, but the risk is far lower than that of smoking tobacco. Overall, 20% of smokers develop lung cancer. This is largely due to individual differences in carcinogen metabolic activation and detoxification.

The prevalence of lung cancer is much higher in men than in women, but this is largely due to differences in tobacco smoking and temporal changes in the pattern of cigarette smoking. Ethnicity, sex, and socioeconomic status have been shown to act as distinct risk factors for lung cancer. In the UK, there is a higher incidence among white males than among any other group; this is followed by black males, with Asian males having a significantly lower incidence. White females, however, have a much higher incidence than females from all other ethnic groups. In contrast, in the USA a higher prevalence of lung cancer has been noted among African Americans than among white Americans, although this has been partially attributed to a higher likelihood of the African American group coming from a lower socioeconomic status, which is in itself associated with an increased likelihood of exposure/susceptibility to lung carcinogens such as tobacco. A similar finding of an increased incidence of lung cancer in groups from a lower socioeconomic status has been noted in the UK. A family history of lung cancer is associated with increased risk, and risk increases if more members of a family have a history of lung cancer.

There is a clear link between lung cancer and other respiratory diseases, mainly COPD and lung fibrosis. Smoking is the main cause of COPD and lung cancer, but smokers with COPD and airflow obstruction are at much higher risk of lung cancer. The risk of lung cancer in patients with COPD is two to three times higher than that in patients without COPD. There is a suggestion that airflow obstruction due to asthma also increases the risk of lung cancer.

3. How should patients with known risk factor(s) for lung cancer be monitored?

People at high risk of lung cancer have been shown to benefit from screening for lung cancer. Currently most (approximately 80%) patients with lung cancer present with advanced stage incurable disease. Early stage disease (stage I, II, and IIIA) can be cured with surgical resection. The overall 5 year survival rates in this group are 50% compared with 5% for advanced lung cancer. Moreover, 5 year survival is much higher in patients with stage I lung cancer (up to 80%) than in those with stage IIIA cancer (40%). Thus identification of lung cancer at an early stage in high-risk people can save lives.

Previous attempts at lung cancer screening with chest x-ray and/or sputum cytology were not successful. However, recent trials using low-dose CT scans of the chest have shown that it is possible to diagnose more patients with early disease, improve chances of curative surgery, and reduce mortality. Patient selection for screening was based on known risk factors such as age, duration of smoking, ethnicity, and economic status. The National Lung Screening Trial (NLST) screened 50 000 people with no symptoms but who smoked 20–30 cigarettes a day, and found that it reduced the number of people who died from lung cancer. A similar trial from the Netherlands and Belgium (the Nelson Trial) was successful in identifying early lung cancer and improving mortality. These findings have been confirmed by the UK Lung Screening Trial in current and ex-smokers. The US Preventive Services Task Force board recommends a yearly low-dose CT scan for people aged 55–80 years who have a history of heavy smoking (30 pack-years or more) and are current smokers or ex-smokers who have stopped within the last 15 years.

Some of the main concerns raised about annual screening with CT scans include the risk of false positive results and the associated unnecessary anxiety in patients found not to have lung cancer, an overdiagnosis of lung cancers in patients deemed not suitable for intervention in the first place, and the subsequent financial and emotional burden of possibly inappropriate and unnecessary further investigations being undertaken in cases with initially falsely suspicious results. Furthermore, screening with CT scans also exposes patients to a possible unwarranted risk of radiation from frequent CT scanning, which is also a risk factor for cancer.

Follow-up and outcome

The patient's case, including her histological findings, were rediscussed at the lung cancer MDT meeting, where it was agreed that she should meet with the oncology team for further assessment. She was subsequently reviewed in their outpatient clinic and commenced first-line chemotherapy with pemetrexed and cisplatin. She received four cycles of chemotherapy, to which she responded well and has remained stable with ongoing follow-up.

Further reading

Alberg AJ, Brock MV, Ford JG, Samet JM, Spivack SD. Epidemiology of Lung Cancer: Diagnosis and Management of Lung Cancer, 3rd ed: American College of Chest Physicians evidence-based clinical practice guidelines. Chest. 2013 May;**143**(5 Suppl):e1S–e29S.

Gould MK. Clinical practice. Lung-cancer screening with low-dose computed tomography. N Engl J Med. 2014 Nov 6;**371**(19):1813–20.

Case 3

Incidental solitary pulmonary nodule in an Afro-Caribbean female ex-smoker

Adam Ainley, Sashin Kaneria,
and Himender Makker

Case history

A 58 year old Afro-Caribbean female was referred to the respiratory clinic because of an incidental nodule found on chest x-ray (Fig. 3.1) when she presented to an accident and emergency department with angina related chest pain. She had no symptoms of breathlessness, cough, fever, or night sweats. She had a past medical history of ischaemic heart disease, hypertension, osteoporosis, and a benign right-sided breast lump. She was an ex-smoker with a 5 pack-year history, having stopped smoking 10 years previously. Physical examination showed no abnormality and lung function tests were normal with an FEV_1 of 2.03 L (95% of predicted) and an FVC of 2.56 L (99% of predicted). She had a CT chest scan (Fig. 3.2).

Questions

1. What does the CT scan show?
2. What are the guidelines for the management of incidental pulmonary nodule(s)?
3. How would you investigate this patient, who has a pulmonary nodule of >8 mm on CT scan and a high (>10%) risk of malignancy?

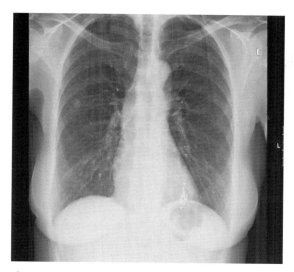

Fig. 3.1 Chest x-ray.

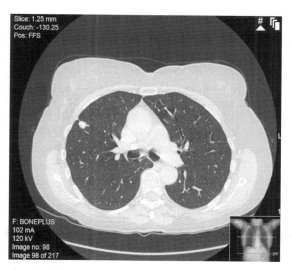

Fig. 3.2 CT chest.

Answers

1. What does the CT scan show?

There is a 1.3 cm nodule in the right mid-zone. The remainder of the lungs and the hila are within normal limits. The nodule shows calcification and most probably represents an old granuloma. There are two additional smaller nodules in the right lung also with evident calcification. The small mediastinal lymph nodes can be seen but are not of significant size.

Incidental pulmonary nodules on CT scans of the chest are common. Their prevalence depends on the geographical background of the population: it is much higher (35%) in countries with a high prevalence of granulomatous diseases such as Asia and Africa but is not so high in the UK (14%). Some of these nodules turn out to be early lung cancer. The prevalence of lung cancer in incidental nodules varies according to the demographic characteristics and smoking prevalence in the population: 2% in North America compared with 0.5% in Asia. The prevalence of pulmonary nodules is much higher in the lung cancer screening population (33%) than in those with incidental nodules (13%), but the prevalence of lung cancer (1.5%) appears to be similar to that in the population with incidental nodules. A much higher prevalence of pulmonary nodules and cancer has been reported in patients with cancer at either staging or follow-up. It is recommended that the route of identification of pulmonary nodules—incidental, screening for lung cancer, or cancer staging—should not guide further management.

Pulmonary nodules may present as either a single nodule or as multiple nodules and may or may not be associated with other abnormalities such as mediastinal or hilar lymphadenopathy. A solitary pulmonary nodule is defined as a rounded lesion surrounded by normal pulmonary parenchyma and without any other abnormalities. It is important to characterize and investigate incidental pulmonary nodules accurately as some of these nodules represent early bronchogenic carcinoma. The 5 year survival rate for resection of lung cancer nodules can be as high as 80% compared with 5–8% in patients with advanced lung cancer. Depending on nodule density, pulmonary nodules are divided into solid nodules, i.e. nodules obscuring the underlying bronchial structures, or subsolid nodules; subsolid nodules are further divided into part solid nodules or pure ground-glass nodules.

Some radiological features are helpful in suggesting a benign process. The presence of calcification within a nodule is often suggestive of a granuloma, whereas low density may indicate fat composition. Similarly, a peripheral perifissural or subpleural nodule of triangular appearance of <10 mm is likely to represent an intrapulmonary lymph node. Finally, nodules of <5 mm are likely to be benign and do not require further follow-up.

In addition to radiological findings of the nodule, clinical predictors such as age and smoking are also taken into consideration for predicting the likelihood of a nodule being an early cancer and the requirement for further follow-up and management.

2. What are the guidelines for the management of incidental pulmonary nodule(s)?

The two guidelines currently in use are the Fleischner Society guidelines, initially published in 2005 and updated in 2017, and the British Thoracic Society (BTS) guidelines, published in 2015.

These guidelines use nodule characteristics such as size, shape, and density in addition to clinical features—history of smoking, age, and gender—to identify the risk of lung cancer and to guide further management. Since CT scans are able to detect nodules of even a few millimetres in size, establishing nodule size to predict the risk for lung cancer has been a major challenge. The findings of recent low-dose CT scan lung cancer screening trials have been extremely helpful to guide not only the size but also the density of nodules.

Although the radiological features of a nodule—size, shape, density, and location—are helpful in predicting the risk of malignancy, the addition of clinical risk factors for lung cancer—age, smoking history, previous history of cancer, or family history of cancer—to the prediction model improves the accuracy of predicting malignancy in a nodule. Among various studies using a combination of clinical and radiological features to predict malignancy, the BTS guidelines recommend the use of the Brock University model. This model found an older age, female sex, a family history of lung cancer, emphysema, a larger nodule size, an upper lobe nodule location, paraneoplastic sensory neuronopathy type, lower nodule count, and spiculation to be predictors for malignancy when applied to a large lung cancer screening cohort.

BTS guidelines recommend following up solid pulmonary nodules of ≥5 mm only. CT surveillance is recommended for people with nodules of ≥5 mm and <8 mm in maximum diameter. For nodules of ≥8 mm in maximum diameter additional clinical features of age and cigarette smoking should be used to determine the risk of lung cancer. BTS guidelines recommend further management of nodules of ≥8 mm guided by the application of the Brock University model—this recommends CT surveillance for 2 years in patients with <10% risk of lung cancer and PET-CT scan if the risk is ≥10%.

No CT scan surveillance or follow-up is recommended for nodules of <5 mm, whether solid or subsolid. For people with subsolid nodules of ≥5 mm a further CT scan at 3 months is recommended to identify whether the nodule has resolved, altered, or grown. Patients with a stable nodule at 3 months require further assessment of malignancy in the nodule and application of the Brock Model. Subsequently if there is a <10% risk of malignancy, surveillance CT scanning at 1, 2, and 4 years is recommended, whereas for patients with a higher risk of malignancy of >10% further investigation such as image-guided biopsy is recommended.

The Fleischner Society guidelines were first published in 2005. The extensively revised second edition of the guidelines was published in 2017 in light of information and evidence from lung cancer screening trials. These guidelines apply to patients who are at least 35 years old with nodules detected incidentally on CT scan and do not apply to patients with nodules detected on lung cancer screening. Similarly, these guidelines are not recommended for patients who are known to have primary cancers and a risk of metastasis or for patients who are immunocompromised and at risk of infections. Similar to the BTS guidelines the size of the nodule is one of the major factors guiding further management. The minimum threshold size for recommending follow-up is based on cancer risk in a nodule of 1% or greater. Instead of <4 mm, the threshold is <6 mm for solid nodules. In addition to nodule size and density, clinical risk factors—smoking, exposure to carcinogens, emphysema, fibrosis, upper lobe location, family history of lung cancer, age, and gender—have been recommended to categorize lung cancer risk as low, intermediate, or high. The high-risk category (older age, heavy smoking, larger nodule size, irregular or spiculated margin, and upper lobe location) have a >65% risk of a nodule being cancerous. The low-risk patients (younger age, less smoking, and smaller nodule size with clear margins located in an area other than the upper lobe) have a lower risk of <5% of cancer.

Single or multiple nodules of <6 mm, solid or subsolid (part solid or ground glass), in patients with a low lung cancer risk do not require follow-up. An optional CT scan at 12 months is recommended in patients with a solid nodule and a high lung cancer risk. In patients with multiple nodules, an infectious cause should be considered.

Single or multiple nodules of 6–8 mm require CT surveillance: 2 years for a solid nodule and a longer follow-up of 5 years for subsolid nodules. An earlier CT scan at 3 months is recommended in patients with a solid nodule at high risk of lung cancer with a view to performing further PET-CT scans and tissue sampling should any growth be noted. A solid nodule that is stable for 2 years is considered to be benign in nature. In patients with multiple nodules the risk of lung cancer increases with increasing number of nodules from one to five and subsequently decreases with a further increase in the number of nodules thereafter. The most suspicious nodule should be used to guide management. These are more likely to represent pulmonary metastasis.

Nodules of >8 mm require a repeat CT scan at 3 months with a view to performing a further PET-CT scan and tissue sampling.

3. How would you investigate this patient, who has a pulmonary nodule of >8 mm on CT scan and a high (>10%) risk of malignancy?

The possible options are CT surveillance, CT-directed biopsy, or surgical excision.

Guidelines recommend PET-CT scan to guide further management. Overall, PET scanning has good sensitivity and specificity for determining malignancy in a nodule of ≥10 mm but the evidence is limited for nodules of <10 mm. The addition of CT to PET (PET-CT) improves the malignancy risk prediction. Risk prediction very much depends on FDG uptake: it can be defined quantitatively as an absolute standardized uptake value (SUV) or qualitatively on an ordinal scale from absent, faint, moderate to intense. Nodules with an SUV ≥2.5 are highly likely to be malignant, but the possibility of malignancy cannot be excluded if the SUV is <2.5. Since it has proven difficult to exclude malignancy with a single SUV cut-off, BTS guidelines have suggested the qualitative assessment of FDG uptake to establish the risk of malignancy and the requirement for further intervention, and have also suggested Herder's model for predicting malignancy. It is recommended that patients with <10% risk of malignancy should have a surveillance CT scan with further stratification using the Brock model. Those ≥10% and <70% risk of malignancy should have a CT-directed biopsy, and those with ≥70% risk of malignancy should have surgical excision without or without image-guided biopsy.

Further reading

Callister ME et al. British Thoracic Society guidelines for the investigation and management of pulmonary nodules. Thorax. 2015 Aug;**70**(Suppl 2):ii1–ii54.

MacMahon H et al. Guidelines for management of incidental pulmonary nodules detected on CT images: from the Fleischner Society 2017. Radiology. 2017 Jul;**284**(1):228–43.

Case 4

Advanced lung cancer on CT pulmonary angiogram in a patient presenting to an accident and emergency department with chest pain and breathlessness

Adam Ainley and Himender Makker

Case history

A 72 year old Greek Cypriot male presented to an accident and emergency department with a 3 month history of worsening left-sided chest discomfort and increasing shortness of breath on exertion, orthopnoea, and paroxysmal nocturnal dyspnoea. He had a long history of cough productive of white phlegm but no haemoptysis. He was a smoker with a 40 pack-year history. He had a reduced appetite and had lost a stone in weight. He had multiple co-morbidities including type 2 diabetes mellitus, hypertension, COPD, and ischaemic heart disease. He also had a history of resection of bladder carcinoma and abdominal aortic aneurysm repair.

He was hypotensive, tachycardic, and hypoxic on admission. Chest auscultation showed reduced air entry on the left side and bilateral crepitations to mid-zones. Heart sounds were normal. His abdomen was soft, with a large non-tender incisional hernia, and an ileostomy draining clear urine. ECG showed atrial fibrillation with a fast ventricular response but his serum troponin was negative. Rate control and diuresis were commenced. A CT angiogram of the aorta excluded any recurrence of the aneurysm of the thoracic aorta or dissection. However, a soft tissue left upper lobe mass was seen encasing the left main bronchus and left main pulmonary artery, with subsequent segmental collapse (Fig. 4.1). Multiple enlarged lymph nodes were also noted, as well as bilateral adrenal adenoma. The liver was seen to be unremarkable. His case was discussed at the lung cancer MDT meeting and subsequent bronchoscopy undertaken; this revealed a tumour completely obstructing the left main bronchus. Bronchial biopsies obtained were found to be negative for lung cancer but, given that the underlying suspicion of malignancy remained, a right axillary lymph node biopsy was performed, which confirmed a diagnosis of SCLC. He was subsequently seen in the rapid access lung clinic to discuss his ongoing management but declined chemotherapy as he had clinically deteriorated and wanted to avoid any ongoing medical interventions.

Questions

1. How often does lung cancer present as a medical emergency?
2. What are the common respiratory presentations of lung cancer?

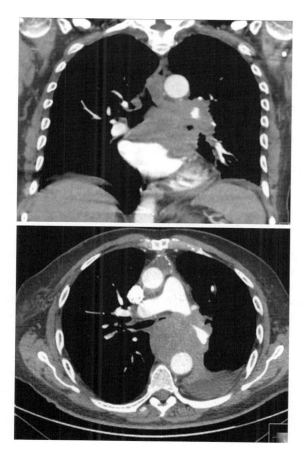

Fig. 4.1 CT chest scan: large left-sided tumour encasing the left main bronchus and occluding the left main pulmonary artery with associated left lower lobe collapse.

Answers

1. How often does lung cancer present as a medical emergency?

Despite rapid access target clinics, 34% of lung cancer patients in the UK are currently diagnosed as an emergency. This figure is significantly higher for lung cancer than for other cancers. Most patients presenting with acute or emergency features of lung cancer have advanced disease. Lung cancer remains one of the most common causes of cancer death: more than one in five cancer deaths are due to lung cancer. The late presentation or emergency presentation of lung cancer is due to a combination of factors. Absence of a screening programme for lung cancer in the UK, despite good evidence that low-dose CT screening reduces mortality by 20%, is likely to be a factor in late and emergency presentations of lung cancer.

2. What are the common respiratory presentations of lung cancer?

Respiratory presentations of lung cancer depend upon the size and site of the tumour. Central lung cancers are more likely to be symptomatic than peripheral tumours. The common presentations of central lung cancer are persistent cough, haemoptysis, shortness of breath, wheeze, and postobstructive pneumonia, whereas peripheral tumours, particularly those involving the pleura, present with chest pain, shortness of breath, and pleural effusion.

Central endobronchial tumours cause persistent cough and more than half of patients have haemoptysis. Haemoptysis is a presenting symptom in 7–10% of patients, occurs during the course of the illness in 30%, and massive haemoptysis (usually due to erosion of blood vessels by the tumour) is the cause of death in up to 3% of patients. It is worth keeping in mind that haemoptysis is also a complication of targeted treatment/immunotherapy for lung cancer with the antigenic agent bevacizumab which is contraindicated in patients with lung cancer who have significant haemoptysis, particularly those with squamous cell carcinoma.

Tracheal and bronchial obstruction occurs in 20–30% of patients with lung cancer. The endobronchial obstruction can progress quite rapidly, leading to respiratory distress and death. It has been suggested that endobronchial central airway obstruction accounts for 40% of lung cancer deaths. These patients have a poor prognosis and survival does not often exceed 1–2 months from point of diagnosis. The treatment of endobronchial obstruction can improve symptoms, lung function tests, and quality of life, and may improve mortality. Central airway obstruction is due to either complete or partial obstruction of the trachea or main bronchus by an endobronchial tumour or extrinsic compression from bulky hilar or mediastinal lymphadenopathy. It mostly occurs in patients with an established diagnosis of lung cancer and causes a progressive increase in breathlessness and respiratory distress. However, this is not an uncommon first presentation of lung cancer. Overall, lung cancer accounts for one-third of patients presenting with central airway obstruction. Main bronchi central airway obstruction causes collapse of the lung and patients present with worsening cough and breathlessness. However, a tracheal tumour may remain undetected until there is critical narrowing of the trachea and patients present with breathlessness and stridor. If not detected and treated early it can rapidly progress into respiratory failure. Early detection of central airway obstruction provides an opportunity for effective palliation of breathlessness and improved quality of life and may improve survival. Urgent imaging and bronchoscopy defines the type of endobronchial obstruction and aids in the selection of the endobronchial procedure required for relief of the obstruction, such as endobronchial laser resection or placement of an endobronchial stent. Relief of an endobronchial obstruction and stabilization of respiratory distress provides an opportunity for further treatment such as external beam radiation or chemotherapy.

A recent study found that about half of patients visited their GP two or more times before an appropriate referral was made. This was despite patients presenting with symptoms that were indicative of lung cancer, such as cough, haemoptysis, chest pain, and back ache. Although the above symptoms are commonly seen among patients with lung cancer, it must also be noted that the majority of patients presenting with the above symptoms to GPs will not have lung cancer, which highlights the difficulties faced in detecting cases based upon symptoms alone.

Further reading

British Lung Foundation. Tackling Emergency Presentation of Lung Cancer: An Expert Working Group Report and Recommendations. London, UK: British Lung Foundation; 2015.

Chen K, Varon J, Wenker O. Malignant airway obstruction: recognition and management. J Emerg Med. 1998:**16**(1):83–92.

Ernst A, Feller-Kopman D, Becher HD, Mehta AC. Central airway obstruction. Am J Respir Crit Care Med. 2004;**169**(12):1278–97.

Case 5

Impaired vision in an ex-smoker

Adam Ainley and Himender Makker

Case history

A 74 year old male presented to an accident and emergency department with a 3 week history of impaired vision. His wife noted that he was frequently bumping into things while walking around the house and had becoming increasingly frail. He had had a chronic dry cough for 6 months and had noted occasional localized lower back pain. His weight and appetite remained stable. He was an ex-smoker, having stopped 4 years previously, with a 50 pack-year smoking history and was known to have COPD.

On neurological examination he had a left-sided homonymous hemianopia. On further clinical examination his breath sounds were reduced at the left lung base and he had mild localized tenderness over the lower thoracic spine.

In light of his symptoms, in addition to the CT head scan a chest x-ray was also undertaken and routine blood tests were performed (Figs 5.1 and 5.2 and Table 5.1).

Questions

1. What do the patient's radiological investigations show?
2. What does the MRI of the brain show?
3. What does the MRI of the spine show?
4. Are the patient's serum electrolytes relevant in the context of his clinical presentation?
5. What additional tests would you request, if any, to further investigate the cause of the patient's electrolyte changes?

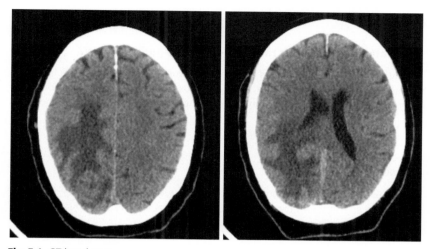

Fig. 5.1 CT head scan.

Table 5.1 Haematology and serum biochemistry results

White cell count	10.0×10^9/L	Serum potassium	5.1 mmol/L
Neutrophil count	5.4×10^9/L	Serum sodium	127 mmol/L
Haemoglobin	13.8 g/L	Creatinine	129 µmol/L
Platelet count	142×10^9/L	Urea	7.6 mmol/L
INR	1.0	Calcium	2.43 mmol/L

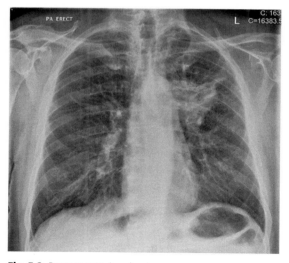

Fig. 5.2 Posteroanterior chest x-ray.

Answers

1. What do the patient's radiological investigations show?

The patient's CT head scan shows a 3 cm focal lesion within the right parietal region with associated vasogenic oedema, raising the possibility of a neoplastic lesion, especially in the context of his chest x-ray, which shows a focal lesion in the left upper lobe.

Case history continued

The patient's CT head scan and chest x-ray were reviewed by the on-call medical team and an MRI of his brain and spine were requested because of his localized back pains (Figs 5.3 and 5.4).

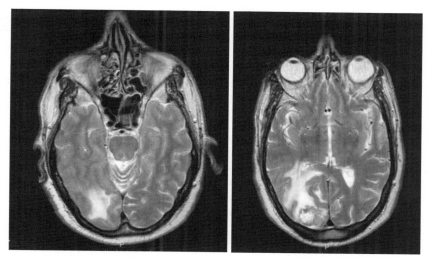

Fig. 5.3 MRI brain.

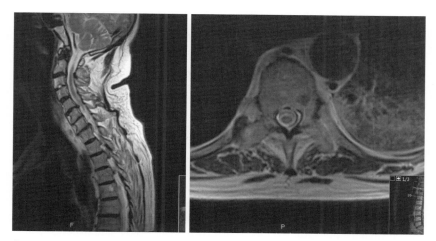

Fig. 5.4 MRI of the thoracic spine.

2. What does the MRI of the brain show?

The MRI of the patient's brain confirmed a 2.6 cm lesion with predominantly per- ipheral enhancement within the juxtacortical white matter of the right posterior parietal/occipital region with significant surrounding oedema, effacement of the ad- jacent sulci, and compression of the posterior horn of the right lateral ventricle. The oedema extended into the majority of the right occipital and parietal lobes. Overall, the findings were of cerebral metastasis.

Brain metastasis. Lung cancer is the most common cause of metastatic brain lesions. Brain metastasis is more common in squamous cell lung cancer than in any other type of NSCLC. Brain metastasis is a presenting feature in 7–10% of patients with NSCLC and develops in 20–30% of patients during the course of illness. Overall, there has been an increase in the incidence of brain metastases associated with lung cancer. This partially reflects use of better imaging/more frequent use of routine imaging techniques and improvement in survival in patients with lung cancer with improved systemic therapies. It is important to note that brain metastases cannot be evaluated reliably using PET-CT due to the intense background FDG uptake. While patients with brain metastases used to have a poor prognosis (1–3 months survival), there has been an improvement in survival (up to 8–9 months) with sys- temic chemotherapy, stereotactic brain surgery, and newer immunotherapy.

3. What does the MRI of the spine show?

The MRI of the patient's thoracic spine shows a sclerotic lesion confined to the T10 vertebral body, in keeping with a metastatic deposit. There was no extension into the vertebral canal or compromise of the spinal cord, and both vertebral body height and alignment were otherwise normal throughout.

Bone metastasis. Lung cancer is the third most common cause of bony metastases following breast and prostate cancer. At least one-third of patients develop bony metastases during the course of their illness. In more than half of patients metastases are present at the time of diagnosis or are a presenting feature. They are frequently multiple and osteolytic and are mostly seen in the spine and pelvic bones. However, bony metastases may be asymptomatic at the time of diagnosis. Most patients present with skeletal-related events (SREs) during the course of their illness and the frequent SREs include pathological fracture, spinal cord compression, and hypercalcaemia. These events may cause intractable pain and affect the patient's quality of life. Overall, patients with SREs at presentation tend to have a worse prognosis than those who develop SREs after diagnosis of metastatic bone disease. The first SRE may occur up to 7 months after detection of bony metastasis. The prognosis for patients with SREs is poorer than for those without SREs, and a scoring system has been suggested to es- timate the survival of patients with bony metastases. Patients score 1 for each feature present, such as age >65 years, non-adenocarcinoma histology, Eastern Cooperative Oncology Group (ECOG) performance status of <2, and type of bone metastases. Patients with a score of ≥2 have a worse prognosis.

There is some evidence that patients with bony metastases treated with TKIs or bevacizumab as a first-line treatment have better survival than those treated with chemotherapy. A newer type of immunotherapy treatment, denosumab, is a new bone-targeted therapy, and success has been documented in patients with bony metastases arising from solid tumours including NSCLC.

4. Are the patient's serum electrolytes relevant in the context of his clinical presentation?

The presence of hyponatraemia (sodium, 127 mmol/L; normal range 135–145 mmol/L) with normal potassium, urea, and electrolyte levels may suggest a diagnosis of the syndrome of inappropriate antidiuretic hormone (SIADH), especially in the context of suspected metastatic lung cancer.

5. What additional tests would you request, if any, to further investigate the cause of the patient's electrolyte changes?

Case history continued

In light of the patient's existing clinical presentation and investigations, paired osmolalities, urinary sodium, and blood glucose were requested, as shown in Table 5.2, and an endocrinology opinion was sought.

The results shown in Table 5.2 demonstrate a low plasma osmolality (< 280 mOsmol/kg) with a high urine osmolality (>100 mOsmol/kg) and raised urinary sodium (>20 mmol/L). These findings are consistent with a diagnosis of SIADH. Although SIADH can be caused by a wide variety of conditions in the context of a patient with metastatic lung cancer, a paraneoplastic process should be suspected.

Hyponatraemia in lung cancer. A serum sodium of <135 mmol/L is a common finding in patients with lung cancer either at the time of diagnosis or during the

Table 5.2 Further investigation results

Serum osmolality	270 mOsmol/kg
Urine osmolality	796 mOsmol/kg
Urinary sodium	40 mmol/L
Capillary blood glucose	6.9 mmol/L

course of the illness. It is often asymptomatic, but may cause neurological symptoms depending upon the degree of severity. It is usually caused by SIADH, either due to ectopic production of arginine vasopressin (AVP) by tumours (mostly SCLC) or as a side effect of anticancer and palliative medications. Approximately 25% of patients with SCLC develop hyponatraemia during the course of their illness and it is a poor prognostic factor. However, hyponatraemia in patients with lung cancer may also be due to other factors such as hypervolaemia secondary to diarrhoea and vomiting. These patients often have a high plasma and low urine osmolality and low urinary sodium.

An endocrinology opinion should be sought to help optimize further management and investigation. Treatment options for patients with hyponatraemia due to inappropriate antidiuretic hormone secretions may include hypertonic saline for acutely symptomatic patients, fluid restriction for chronic asymptomatic patients, and selective AVP receptor 2 (V2)-receptor antagonists, e.g. tolvaptan, if fluid restriction is ineffective.

Follow-up and outcome

The patient's CT chest scan revealed a 7.2 cm mass in the left upper lobe of the lung extending into the mediastinum, and bronchoscopy revealed an intraluminal lesion. Biopsies confirmed a moderate to poorly differentiated squamous cell carcinoma. His World Health Organization (WHO) performance status was 1–2. He was on dexamethasone 8 mg twice a day and a proton-pump inhibitor for gastric protection. Endocrinologists confirmed a diagnosis of SIADH and recommended fluid restriction. He was also discussed at the neurosurgery MDT meeting. He was reviewed by the oncology team and he expressed a wish to have only conservative interventions. A referral to the Macmillan services and community hospice was requested.

Further reading

Ali A, Goffin JR, Arnold A, Ellis PM. Survival of patients with non-small-cell lung cancer after a diagnosis of brain metastases. Curr Oncol. 2013 Aug;**20**(4):e300–6.

Castillo JJ, Vincent M, Justice E. Diagnosis and management of hyponatremia in cancer patients. Oncologist. 2012;**17**(6):756–65.

Santini D et al. Natural history of non-small-cell lung cancer with bone metastases. Sci Rep. 2015 Dec 22;**5**:18670.

Case 6

Late recurrence or second primary lung cancer?

Adam Ainley and Himender Makker

Case history

A 69 year old female who had had a wedge resection for a stage I right upper lobe adenocarcinoma 8 years previously was referred by her GP to the respiratory clinic because of right apical chest wall pain and a dry cough. She denied any breathlessness and had no weight loss or reduced appetite. Her WHO performance status was 1. She was an ex-tobacco smoker of 15 pack-years, having stopped smoking 10 years previously. She had a strong family history of cancer: her mother had pancreatic carcinoma, one sister had ovarian carcinoma, and another sister had breast cancer. Her brother was recently diagnosed with oesophageal cancer.

There was no obvious abnormality on examination but chest x-ray showed a right upper zone shadow. A CT scan of her chest, abdomen, and pelvis confirmed a 3.6 cm right upper lobe mass adjacent to the right oblique fissure, a 5 mm nodular opacity in the right lower lobe, a small to moderate size pericardial effusion, and a 2.3 cm mediastinal lymph node adjacent to the left superior pulmonary vein with evidence of necrosis. A left adrenal lobulated mass was also noted.

Questions

1. How would you investigate this patient further?
2. What does this patient's PET-CT scan demonstrate?
3. Further to the results of the PET-CT scan what further investigations would you consider?
4. How common is recurrence of lung cancer after curative surgical resection?
5. How common is late recurrence of lung cancer after curative resection of stage I NSCLC?
6. What are the predictors of recurrence after curative surgical resection?
7. How would you manage recurrence of lung cancer?

Answers

1. How would you investigate this patient further?

The patient should be investigated in a similar fashion to all new patients with suspected lung cancer: confirmation of the histological diagnosis with EBUS/CT-directed biopsy and accurate staging with EBUS/PET-CT.

Case history continued

After reviewing her staging CT scan, a PET-CT was requested (Fig. 6.1).

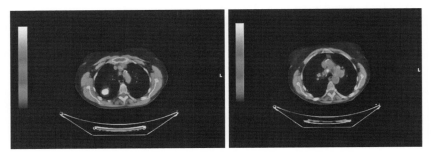

Fig. 6.1 PET-CT scan.

2. What does this patient's PET-CT scan demonstrate?

There is an FDG-avid right upper lobe lesion with increased uptake in the mediastinal lymph nodes.

Case history continued

The right upper lobe mass was reported to have an SUV$_{max}$ of 24.6. There were multiple FDG-avid ipsilateral and contralateral mediastinal lymph nodes. The liver, spleen, and adrenal glands showed no uptake.

3. Further to the results of the PET-CT scan what further investigations would you consider?

The clinical history and results of the radiological investigations so far are in keeping with a suspected underlying malignant process. As such the main aim of any further investigation would be to obtain tissue in order to gain histological evidence for further confirmation of the diagnosis.

Case history continued

In view of the PET-CT findings the patient had a CT-guided biopsy of the primary lesion, which confirmed that the lung parenchyma was infiltrated by a poorly differentiated NSCLC. On immunohistochemistry (IHC) the tumour stained positive with mucin stain. IHC results for AE1/3, 34BE12, TTF-1, CK7, and carcinoembryonic antigen (CEA) were all positive. CK5/6, WT-1, calretinin, and p63 were all negative, with BerEp4 non-contributory. In order to further assess the lymph nodes seen on PET-CT an EBUS-guided bronchoscopy was undertaken with lymph node biopsies taken from station 4R. Histologically fragments of lymphoid tissue were present that were associated with anthracotic pigment, although no evidence of malignancy was identified. The overall appearances were in keeping with an adenocarcinoma.

4. How common is recurrence of lung cancer after curative surgical resection?

Despite complete curative resection 30–75% of lung cancers recur. The high rate of recurrence is thought to be due to the inability of current diagnostic and imaging techniques to detect occult micrometastatic disease. Most recurrences (80%) occur during the first 2 years after surgical resection and often involve distant metastasis. The risk of recurrence gradually diminishes over a 5 year period with virtually no recurrences seen after 5 years. Local recurrences are less common and most often occur during the first year, peaking at 9 months after surgery, followed by two smaller peaks at the end of the second and fourth year post resection. However, the incidence of a new second primary lesion is approximately 2% per year, and the risk increases even after 5 years (Fig. 6.2).

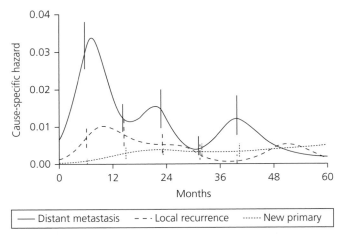

Fig. 6.2 Cause-specific hazard rate estimates for local recurrence, distant metastasis, and second primary in 1506 patients undergoing surgery with curative intent for early-stage non-small-cell cancer. Reprinted from Demicheli R, et al Recurrence dynamics for non-small-cell lung cancer: effect of surgery on the development of metastases. *J Thorac Oncol* 2012;7:723–30 with permission from Elsevier.

5. How common is late recurrence of lung cancer after curative resection of stage I NSCLC?

Overall 5 year survival in stage I resected lung cancer varies from 80% to 93%. However, late recurrences after the first 5 years of cancer-free survival are not uncommon. A late recurrence rate of 4.8% has been reported in stage IA resected NSCLC, with an almost equal split for locoregional recurrences and distant metastasis. Late recurrences are more likely to occur in patients who had adenocarcinoma and evidence of vascular invasion in the resected tumour. It has been suggested that the current practice of 5 years of postresection surveillance may not capture all patients who subsequently develop disease recurrence.

6. What are the predictors of recurrence after curative surgical resection?

TNM staging remains the main predictor of recurrence, with much higher rates in stage IIIA than in stage I resected lung cancer. However, there is a huge variation in recurrence even among patients within the same stage of lung cancer. Numerous attempts have been made to identify patients at higher risk of recurrence based on tumour characteristics—lymphatic permeation, pleural invasion, poor histological differentiation, and vascular and visceral invasion are associated with a higher risk of recurrence. Various tumour markers have also been identified to help predict recurrence.

Clinical and radiological features have also been used to guide predictions of recurrence. Features such as symptoms and WHO performance status have been shown to be consistent predictors of disease-free survival whereas a higher FDG uptake on PET scan (SUV) has been associated with an increased risk of recurrence.

It is recommended that most patients should have regular surveillance for detection of early recurrence. Various strategies have been suggested, including clinical review, chest x-ray, and CT scan. Although most guidelines agree on the value of ongoing clinical review for a duration of 5 years, the role of CT follow-up has mostly superseded routine chest x-ray. American College of Chest Physicians guidelines (2013) recommend CT surveillance every 6 months for the first 2 years and on an annual basis thereafter. This recommendation was based upon large but uncontrolled retrospective studies, which showed better 5 year survival in patients who were followed up with CT scan than in those who were followed up with chest x-ray. CT surveillance is also more likely to help with the early detection of a second primary. There is no evidence yet to show whether more sophisticated imaging techniques such as PET-CT or biochemical methods using the detection of molecular markers in blood or sputum improve outcome.

7. How would you manage recurrence of lung cancer?

Management of recurrence should be based on histological type and staging, similar to an initial presentation of lung cancer. However, relatively few patients with local recurrence or a second primary are well enough for a second curative surgical resection, but there is an increasing role for curative stereotactic ablative radiotherapy (SABR) resection.

Follow-up and outcome

The patient was discussed at the lung cancer MDT meeting, where it was agreed that she had a likely recurrence of adenocarcinoma. However, the spread of disease was more advanced than her initial episode and her malignancy was deemed inoperable. Her EGFR status was negative. As her performance status was good the oncologists reviewed her and palliative chemotherapy was recommended.

Further reading

Colt HG, Murgu SD, Korst RJ, Slatore CG, Unger M, Quadrelli S. Follow-up and surveillance of the patient with lung cancer after curative-intent therapy: Diagnosis and management of lung cancer, 3rd ed: American College of Chest Physicians evidence-based clinical practice guidelines. Chest. 2013 May;**143**(5 Suppl):e437S–e454S.

Maeda R, Yoshida J, Ishii G, Aokage K, Hishida T, Nishimura M, Nishiwaki Y, Nagai K. Long-term outcome and late recurrence in patients with completely resected stage IA non-small cell lung cancer. J Thorac Oncol. 2010 Aug;5(8):1246–50.

Matsumura Y et al. Early and late recurrence after intentional limited resection for cT1aN0M0, non-small cell lung cancer: from a multi-institutional, retrospective analysis in Japan. Interact Cardiovasc Thorac Surg. 2016 Sep;23(3):444–9.

van Meerbeeck JP, Sirimsi H. Cons: long-term CT-scan follow-up is not the standard of care in patients curatively treated for an early stage non-small cell lung cancer. Transl Lung Cancer Res. 2015 Aug;4(4):479–83.

Case 7

Endobronchial tumour in a smoker with a history of lymphoma

Adam Ainley, Bryan Sheinman, and Himender Makker

Case history

A 70 year old female with a complex past medical history was referred to the lung cancer clinic having presented acutely to an accident and emergency department with a 3 month history of worsening breathlessness on exertion and a 1 month history of intermittent cough associated with episodes of haemoptysis. She reported a 1 week history of chest pain that had become more persistent, prompting her attendance at the accident and emergency department. She had recently received a 1 week course of antibiotics from her GP, which had not resolved her symptoms. The antibiotics were prescribed because of her abnormal chest x-ray shown in Fig. 7.1.

On review in the accident and emergency department her symptoms were thought to be suggestive of a pulmonary embolus and a CT pulmonary angiogram was arranged (Fig. 7.2). No pulmonary embolus was found, but a focal abnormality was seen in the left upper lobe, prompting a discussion with the respiratory team. The respiratory team arranged to see her the next day in the rapid access lung cancer clinic.

When seen in the lung cancer clinic the patient reported no additional symptoms and denied any constitutional symptoms. She was an ex-tobacco smoker of 40 pack-years, but had given up 20 years previously. She had been diagnosed with, and received chemotherapy for, B-cell lymphoma 11 years previously with no relapse. Her husband died of lung cancer 5 years previously, having been a heavy tobacco smoker.

On examination, breath sounds were reduced at the left base with bronchial breathing at the left apex. There was no palpable lymphadenopathy and abdominal examination was unremarkable. The patient's WHO performance status was 1.

Questions

1. In light of this patient's initial findings, which investigation would you request next in order to confirm a suspected underlying pulmonary malignancy?

2. Is there any value in obtaining samples of sputum given the patient's intermittent cough?

3. What is the role of bronchoscopy in obtaining a diagnosis of lung cancer?

4. What techniques are useful during bronchoscopy in the diagnosis of lung cancer?

5. Are all patients suitable for bronchoscopy and what assessments need to be undertaken?

6. In light of the patient's clinical, radiological, and histological findings what clinical staging would you give this female?

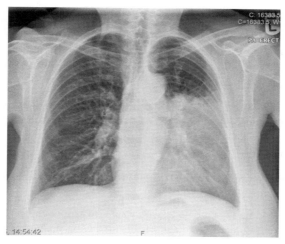

Fig. 7.1 Chest x-ray of a 70 year old female with a 3 month history of worsening breathlessness, a 1 month history of cough, and a 1 week history of chest pain.

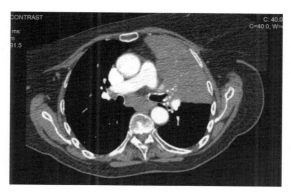

Fig. 7.2 CT pulmonary angiogram showing left upper lobe collapse consolidation.

Answers

1. In light of this patient's initial findings, which investigation would you request next in order to confirm a suspected underlying pulmonary malignancy?

Given the patient's good performance status and left upper lobe collapse/consolidation, bronchoscopy should be performed in addition to a full, staging, contrast-enhanced CT of the chest and abdomen.

2. Is there any value in obtaining samples of sputum given the patient's intermittent cough?

Although it would be appropriate to send a sputum sample for further cytological and microbiological analysis a diagnosis of underlying malignancy could not be excluded by a negative sample. Sputum cytology is only recommended as an investigation when the patient is considered unsuitable for, or is unwilling to undergo, any other interventions. This recommendation is based upon the varying results of studies which have demonstrated vastly different diagnostic yields using sputum samples. The overall sensitivity of sputum cytology for lung cancer is between 42% and 97%, with a specificity ranging from 68% to 100%. Factors that are thought to increase the likelihood of sputum cytology being positive include the sample being bloody, central tumour location, squamous cell type, and if the tumour is large (>2.4 cm). When sputum cytology is undertaken, it is suggested that at least three specimens are obtained in order to increase the diagnostic yield.

Case history continued

At bronchoscopy a large endobronchial mass lesion was found in the left main bronchus with almost 60% occlusion (Fig. 7.3). There was evidence of distal bleeding. During the procedure an endobronchial needle biopsy, brushings, and washings were taken.

3. What is the role of bronchoscopy in obtaining a diagnosis of lung cancer?

It is recommended that a CT of the thorax should be undertaken prior to bronchoscopy for accurate localization of the site of sampling. Direct exploration of the bronchial tree via conventional flexible bronchoscopy (FB) is the most useful and is indicated when a central (endobronchial) lesion has been seen during radiological investigations or is clinically suspected. In addition to allowing direct visualization of the bronchial tree and allowing the localization of any abnormalities, samples

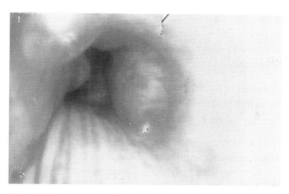

Fig. 7.3 Tumour invading the left main bronchus.

can also be taken to confirm both a cytological and histological diagnosis and to undertake further molecular analysis. Obtaining a tissue-based diagnosis is a vital step in managing patients with lung carcinoma and helps to determine the potential management options.

While FB remains the first-line investigation for centrally based lesions, newer, complementary techniques have optimized the procedure to improve detection and sampling of more peripheral lesions. Advanced techniques such as radial-endobronchial ultrasound (R-EBUS) and electromagnetic navigation (EMN) utilize imaging facilities to localize more peripheral lesions and are recommended when lesions are more difficult to reach or visualize directly using the conventional approach. However, both procedures require specialist equipment and expertise and are not yet widely utilized in the UK currently. When a central lesion is not visible bronchoscopically or is also associated with lymphadenopathy, EBUS has a vital role in obtaining a diagnosis and staging of disease. [This is discussed later in this section.]

4. What techniques are useful during bronchoscopy in the diagnosis of lung cancer?

At bronchoscopy a number of sampling techniques can be undertaken, including bronchial brushings, washings/lavage, and endobronchial or transbronchial needle biopsy, to confirm a histological/cytological diagnosis. Tissue biopsy is the optimal method, providing overall sensitivity of around 80% compared with lower sensitivities of both brushings and washings (60% and 50%, respectively). However, it is recommended that all sample modalities be used when possible to increase the overall diagnostic yield, including five biopsy samples. It is recommended that bronchoscopy units have a diagnostic yield of 85% when an endobronchial tumour has been directly visualized.

When peripheral lesions are present, the size of the lesion itself has been shown to affect the diagnostic ability of bronchoscopic techniques. In such circumstances imaging-guided methods such as R-EBUS and EMN have been shown to increase the sensitivity by 20%. EMN in addition to EBUS has been shown to have a diagnostic yield of around 90%. However, even with these methods, the overall diagnostic yield is reduced when target lesions are smaller than 20 mm, when sensitivity is around 56% compared with 78% in larger lesions.

5. Are all patients suitable for bronchoscopy and what assessments need to be undertaken?

Bronchoscopy is a relatively well-tolerated procedure with serious complications in 1.1% of patients undergoing the procedure and an overall mortality of 0.02%. However, it is recommended that the least invasive method of obtaining a tissue diagnosis be undertaken and, ideally, management should be guided by the local lung cancer MDT to ensure that it will add to the potential decision-making without adding any undue risk to the patient. Fitness for the procedure should take into account: the co-morbidities of the patient, in particular any underlying lung diseases, risk of bleeding, and ability to tolerate sedation.

Case history continued

In light of the patient's bronchoscopy findings a PET scan was also arranged, as shown in Fig. 7.4.

The case was discussed at the lung cancer MDT meeting, when the following results were reviewed.

The whole body PET-CT was reported as showing a large, highly metabolically active mass lesion measuring 14 × 6.4 cm in the lingula/left upper lobe (SUV$_{max}$ = 15.6). The mass lesion had invaded the left pulmonary hilum, abutted the aortic arch, the pulmonary trunk and the left pulmonary artery, invaded the mediastinum below the aortic arch, and obstructed the left lower lobe and upper lobe bronchi. There were enlarged highly metabolically active subcarinal nodes (the largest measured 2.2 cm in short axis, SUV$_{max}$ = 14.2), a 9 mm left peribronchial node, a 12 mm posterior mediastinal node in the paraoesophageal position, and a string of highly FDG-avid right paratracheal and pretracheal nodes. There was a mildly metabolically active left pleural effusion. Within the liver, there were multiple metastatic deposits: the largest, in segment 7, measured 6.8 × 3.7 cm (SUV$_{max}$ = 11.4).

Within the skeleton, there were multiple metastatic lesions in the right and left iliac blades; in the vertebral bodies of L4, T12, T11, and T10; in the right posterior element of L3; and in the left 7th rib laterally.

The samples taken from the patient's bronchoscopy revealed no organisms or neoplastic cells in her bronchial washing or brushings; however, the needle biopsy showed bronchial mucosa infiltrated by SCLC. Further immunohistochemical analysis was requested.

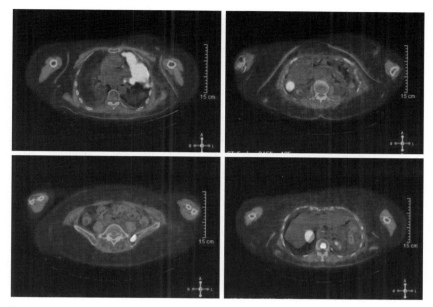

Fig. 7.4 Nuclear Medicine (NM) whole-body PET FDG.

6. In light of the patient's clinical, radiological, and histological findings what clinical staging would you give this female?

The patient was staged as T4N3M1b based upon the seventh lung cancer TNM classification/International Association for the Study of Lung Cancer (IASLC) staging criteria recommended by the Union for International Cancer Control (UICC). Staging reflected the size of the tumour and, most importantly, the associated invasion of the mediastinum and adjacent vessels, multiple mediastinal lymph node involvement, and liver and bone metastases. This would be consistent with a diagnosis of extensive stage SCLC based upon histological use of the previous Veterans Administration Lung Study Group (VALG), which is often still referred to given the simpler two-stage differentiation of the extent of small cell disease.

Follow-up and outcome

Given the patient's performance status she was reviewed by the oncology team, which offered chemotherapy with cisplatin and etoposide. She received four cycles but did not tolerate the fifth. She also received thoracic radiotherapy to help with her chest wall pains. Unfortunately, she developed bilateral pulmonary embolus and her disease progressed despite interventions. The patient was admitted to a hospice 7 months after diagnosis.

Further reading

Eberhardt R, Anantham D, Ernst A, Feller-Kopman D, Herth F. Multimodality bronchoscopic diagnosis of peripheral lung lesions: a randomized controlled trial. Am J Respir Crit Care Med. 2007 Jul;**176**(1):36–41.

Detterbeck FC, Rivera MP, Socinski M, > Rosenman J. Diagnosis and Treatment of Lung Cancer: an Evidence-Based Guide for the Practicing Clinician. Philadelphia, PA: W.B. Saunders; 2001. p. 54.

Du Rand IA et al. BTS guidelines for advanced diagnostic and therapeutic flexible bronchoscopy in adults. Thorax. 2011;**6**(Suppl 3):iii1–iii21.

Hinson KF, Kuper SW. The diagnosis of lung cancer by examination of sputum. Thorax. 1963;**18**:350–3

Risse EK, van't Hof MA, Vooijs GP. Relationship between patient characteristics and sputum cytologic diagnosis of lung cancer. Acta Cytol. 1987;**31**(2):159–65.

Schreiber G, McRory DC. Performance characteristics of different modalities for diagnosis of suspected lung cancer: summary of published evidence. Chest. 2003;**123**(1 Suppl):115S–128S.

Steinfort DP, Khor YH, Manser RL, Irving LB. Radial probe endobronchial ultrasound for the diagnosis of peripheral lung cancer: systematic review and meta-analysis. Eur Respir J. 2011;**37**(4):902–10.

Case 8

Progressive breathlessness associated with a right-sided pleural effusion

Adam Ainley and Himender Makker

Case history

An 83 year old male was referred to the pleural clinic by the acute medical team for management of right-sided pleural effusion. He had become increasingly short of breath over the last few weeks and had noted an occasional dry cough. He denied any chest pains, fevers, or sweats and had not lost weight or his appetite. His WHO performance status was 1. He was a retired painter/decorator but denied any history of asbestos exposure. He was a non-smoker. On examination his S_aO_2 was 95% on room air and there was reduced air entry and dullness on percussion at the right lung base. An ultrasound-guided pleural aspiration showed blood-stained fluid with a protein count of 43 g/dL, lactate dehydrogenase (LDH) of 337 IU/L, and glucose of 4.7 mmol/L. Cytological and microbiological analyses were unremarkable.

Questions

1. What do the patient's pleural fluid results suggest and how useful is the analysis of pleural fluid in obtaining a diagnosis of lung cancer?
2. What does the CT scan show?
3. What additional investigations are recommended to help confirm the diagnosis of lung cancer?
4. How would you assess this patient's suitability for further pleural biopsy?

Answers

1. What do the patient's pleural fluid results suggest and how useful is the analysis of pleural fluid in obtaining a diagnosis of lung cancer?

The patient's pleural fluid results are consistent with an exudative effusion (protein >30 g/dL, fluid–serum protein ratio of >0.5, fluid–serum LDH ratio >0.6, and fluid LDH level than greater than two-thirds of the upper limit of serum LDH) and in the context of his history warrant further investigation.

Although many symptoms associated with pleural effusion are non-specific and may relate to a number of different conditions there is an increased risk of malignancy when the fluid is blood stained and associated with chest discomfort and constitutional symptoms such as weight loss and anorexia.

The presence of a pleural effusion in a patient with suspected lung cancer is an important clinical finding and helps guide overall management. The presence of a pleural effusion provides an alternative site to obtain a tissue diagnosis via less invasive means. It is also useful when staging disease because the presence of a malignant pleural effusion is itself associated with a metastasis stage of M1a and overall indicates stage IV disease.

Pleural fluid cytology should be obtained in all patients with suspected lung cancer when an effusion is found during radiological assessment. Fluid should be obtained via ultrasound-guided aspiration, which both reduces the risk of associated complications and improves the success rate of the procedure. Pleural fluid cytology has a sensitivity of around 70%, and fluid analysis should include immunocytochemistry and molecular testing. There is little evidence on the amount of fluid that should initially be sent; however, there is limited diagnostic benefit versus risk of complications in repeating samples if an initial sample tests negative.

Case history continued

Further to his review in the pleural clinic a CT scan of the patient's chest was performed (Fig. 8.1).

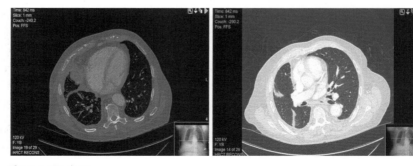

Fig. 8.1 CT chest.

2. What does the CT scan show?

The CT scan demonstrates volume loss and pleural thickening involving the fissures in the right hemithorax with associated basal pleural calcification.

A number of radiological features may be seen that suggest an effusion is more likely to be malignant in nature; these include circumferential pleural thickening, parietal pleural thickening, mediastinal involvement, pleural nodularity, and a thickened diaphragm.

3. What additional investigations are recommended to help confirm the diagnosis of lung cancer?

In patients with a non-diagnostic pleural fluid aspirate and suspected malignancy a pleural biopsy is required. Historically biopsies were carried out blindly using an Abrams needle and the diagnostic yield was poor (57%). However, directly visualized or image-guided pleural biopsies have improved diagnostic yields up to 95%. Pleural biopsy can be undertaken using an image-guided cutting needle using CT or US guidance or directly via thoracoscopy; both methods have relatively equivalent sensitivity and specificity of 90–100%.

4. How would you assess this patient's suitability for further pleural biopsy?

In patients with suspected malignancy where active management is recommended and a pleural fluid aspirate is negative, a pleural biopsy should be undertaken to establish diagnosis and stage the disease. Suitability for the procedure should be discussed at the lung cancer MDT meeting and should take into account the patient's wishes and his/her co-morbidities, including previous pleural procedures, underlying lung conditions, and risk of bleeding. Overall the options are relatively safe and well tolerated. The major complications include bleeding, localized infection, and pneumonia. For image-guided procedures the risk of pneumothorax is greater (3–15%) than for thoracoscopic techniques; however, the risk of overall complications is slightly lower (1–2%) than for thoracoscopic procedures (>2.3%). Surgical options such as video-assisted thoracoscopic surgery (VATS) require a general anaesthetic; as such, patients should be deemed suitable for this additional risk. Overall mortality for surgical options is <0.5%.

Follow-up and outcome

Following further discussion at the lung cancer MDT meeting a VATS biopsy was performed, which showed neoplastic cells. IHC stains were positive for calretinin and CK5/6. The histological and immunological profiles were consistent with a diagnosis of epithelioid malignant mesothelioma. The patient was subsequently referred for port site radiotherapy to the chest wall and further oncological review to discuss additional treatment options.

Further reading

Ferrer J, Roldán J, Teixidor J, Pallisa E, Gich I, Morell F. Predictors of pleural malignancy in patients with pleural effusions undergoing thoracoscopy. Chest. 2005;**127**(3):1012–22.

Harris RJ, Kavuru MS, Mehta AC, Medendorp SV, Wiedemann HP, Kirby TJ, Rice TW. The impact of thoracoscopy on the management of pleural disease. Chest. 1995 Mar;**107**(3):845–52.

Hooper C, Lee YC, Maskell N; BTS Pleural Guideline Group. Investigation of a unilateral pleural effusion in adults: British Thoracic Society pleural disease guideline. Thorax. 2010 Aug;**65**(Suppl 2):ii4e–ii17e.

Leung AN, Müller NL, Miller RR. CT in differential diagnosis of diffuse pleural disease. AJR Am J Roentgenol. 1990 Mar;**154**(3):487–92.

Maskell NA, Gleeson FV, Davies RJ. Standard pleural biopsy versus CT-guided cutting-needle biopsy for diagnosis of malignant disease in pleural effusions: a randomised controlled trial. Lancet. 2003 Apr;**361**(9366):1326–30.

Metintas M, Ak G, Dundar E, Yildirim H, Ozkan R, Kurt E, Erginel S, Alatas F, Metintas S. Medical thoracoscopy vs CT scan-guided Abrams pleural needle biopsy for diagnosis of patients with pleural effusions: a randomised controlled trial. Chest. 2010 Jun;**137**(6):1362–8.

Qureshi NR, Rahman NM, Gleeson FV. Thoracic ultrasound in the diagnosis of malignant pleural effusion. Thorax. 2009 Feb;**64**(2):139–43.

Rahman NM et al. Local anaesthetic thoracoscopy: British Thoracic Society pleural disease guideline. Thorax. 2010 Aug;**65**(Suppl 2):ii54e–ii60e.

Roberts ME, Neville E, Berrisford RG, Antunes G, Ali NJ; BTS Pleural Disease Guideline Group. Management of a malignant pleural effusion: British Thoracic Society pleural disease guideline. Thorax. 2010 Aug;**65**(Suppl 2):ii32e–ii40e.

Tomlinson JR, Sahn SA. Invasive procedures in the diagnosis of pleural disease. Semin Respir Crit Care Med. 1987;**9**(1):30–36.

Case 9

PET-positive right lower lobe mass

Adam Ainley, Sashin Kaneria, and Himender Makker

Case history

An 85 year old female was referred to the lung cancer clinic after a recent hospital admission due to a fall associated with chest discomfort and syncope. During her admission she underwent a CT pulmonary angiogram to exclude pulmonary embolus. Although no embolus was noted, a 3.3 cm right lower lobe lesion was seen (Fig. 9.1). The patient was assessed by a cardiologist, who diagnosed ischaemic heart disease on the basis of coronary angiogram findings of a moderate–severe left anterior descending coronary artery lesion and severe aortic regurgitation. She was being considered for an aortic valve replacement and coronary artery bypass.

The patient had no breathlessness or cough. Although she denied any weight loss or other constitutional symptoms, her son was concerned that she had lost significant weight over the last few weeks. She had osteoporosis but no other medical conditions. The patient was an ex-tobacco smoker of 50 pack-years, having stopped 2 years previously. She was frail with a limited exercise tolerance and a history of recurrent falls. Her WHO performance status was 2. Physical examination did not reveal any focal abnormalities.

Her case was discussed at the lung cancer MDT meeting and, given her performance status, she was referred for PET-CT to stage her disease (Fig. 9.2).

Questions

1. What do Figures 9.1 and 9.2 show?

2. Given her PET-CT findings how would you stage this patient's disease radiologically?

3. How would you obtain a histological diagnosis given this patient's PET-CT results, clinical status, and CT findings?

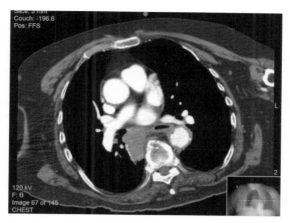

Fig. 9.1 CT chest.

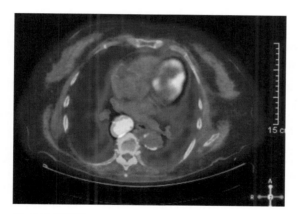

Fig. 9.2 PET-CT.

Answers

1. What do Figures 9.1 and 9.2 show?

A metabolically active (FDG-avid) 4 × 2.4 cm soft tissue mass can be seen in the right lower lobe and is situated at the inferomedial aspect of the right lower lobe bronchus and less than 2 cm from the carina. The mass abuts the prevertebral surface; however, there is no evidence of metabolically active disease involving the skeleton at this site. There was no noted lymphadenopathy or evidence of metabolically active metastatic disease elsewhere.

2. Given her PET-CT findings how would you stage this patient's disease radiologically?

Using the seventh edition of the TNM staging classification the primary lesion is more than 3 cm in size and less than 2 cm in distance from the main carina, which would be classified as stage T3. As there is no evidence of any nodal or metastatic disease the patient would be given a radiological stage of T3N0M0.

3. How would you obtain a histological diagnosis given this patient's PET-CT results, clinical status, and CT findings?

A number of factors need to be considered when deciding the most optimal methods for obtaining a histological diagnosis. Factors including the patient's wishes, his/her premorbid and performance status, and the site and suspected spread of disease must be taken into account.

For all patients who are considered fit for further interventions, histological confirmation of the diagnosis and accurate staging are essential. When a lesion is peripheral and located within the lung parenchyma without lymph node involvement or metastatic disease, surgical options should be considered to provide both a diagnostic and therapeutic option. [This will be discussed in subsequent sections.] When lesions are central or peripheral with associated lymph node involvement, flexible bronchoscopy and EBUS with transbronchial needle aspiration (TBNA) or fine needle aspiration (FNA) should be performed.

TBNA can be used to provide both cytological and histological samples. When possible it is recommended that histological samples are taken in order to provide the best chance of subsequent diagnosis and molecular analysis. The basis for this recommendation is that although FNA has a sensitivity between 88% and 92% it has a higher risk of a false negative diagnosis (approximately 25%) than core biopsies taken for histological analysis using a cutting needle.

Percutaneous (transthoracic) needle biopsy may be undertaken by various radiologically guided methods, including MRI, US, or CT, using an 18–22 gauge cutting needle to obtain a core biopsy. Most biopsies are usually undertaken using CT guidance unless the lesion is close to the chest wall. Percutaneous transthoracic needle sampling is associated with more frequent complications than endoscopic methods. There is a 3% risk of pneumothorax; however, only a minority (2–5%) of patients require a chest tube or catheter. Pneumothorax can be managed in an outpatient setting using a Heimlich valve or thoracic vent. Haemothorax requiring intervention and significant haemoptysis occur in <1% of patients undergoing CT-directed biopsy. These risks are more common in patients older than 60 years, in smokers, and in those with underlying COPD.

Follow-up and outcome

The results of the patient's PET-CT were reviewed at the lung cancer MDT meeting. In light of her performance status, it was thought that she might not tolerate a more invasive procedure such as bronchoscopy. As such she was referred for a CT-guided biopsy. Her subsequent biopsy was reported as demonstrating a moderately differentiated carcinoma with predominantly squamous differentiation. IHC revealed generalized p63 and p40 positivity within the tumour cells while TTF-1 was negative. Focal mucin production was noted, indicating that this was a predominantly squamous cell carcinoma with evidence focally of glandular differentiation.

After her biopsy results were obtained the patient was seen in the lung cancer clinic, where she subsequently declined chemotherapy or radical radiotherapy in light of her progressive decline in functional status, which had deteriorated since her initial referral. She was offered the chance to remain under follow-up for consideration of symptomatic treatment and palliative radiotherapy as required; however, the patient's disease progressed and she was subsequently referred for palliative care input.

Further reading

Detterbeck FC, Rivera MP. Table 4-9. Reliability of needle biopsy of pulmonary nodules to assess the presence of cancer. In: Detterbeck FC, Rivera MP, Socinski M, > Rosenman J, editors. Diagnosis and Treatment of Lung Cancer: an Evidence-Based Guide for the Practicing Clinician. Philadelphia, PA: W.B. Saunders; 2001. p. 57.

Gong Y, Sneige N, Guo M, Hicks ME, Moran CA. Transthoracic fine-needle aspiration vs concurrent core needle biopsy in diagnosis of intrathoracic lesions: a retrospective comparison of diagnostic accuracy. Am J Clin Pathol. 2006 Mar;**125**(3):438–44.

Nicholson T, editor. Recommendations for Cross-sectional Imaging in Cancer Management. Second edition. London, UK: Royal College of Radiologists; 2014.

Schreiber G, McRory DC. Performance characteristics of different modalities for diagnosis of suspected lung cancer: summary of published evidence. Chest. 2003;**123**(1 Suppl):115S–128S.

Wiener RS, Schwartz LM, Woloshin S, Welch HG. Population-based risk for complications after transthoracic needle lung biopsy of a pulmonary nodule: an analysis of discharge records. Ann Intern Med. 2011;**155**(3):137–44.

Zarbo RJ, Fenoglio-Preiser CM. Interinstitutional database for comparison of performance in lung fine-needle aspiration cytology. A College of American Pathologists Q-Probe Study of 5264 cases with histologic correlation. Arch Pathol Lab Med. 1992;**116**(5):463–70.

Case 10

Histology of a right hilar mass in an ex-smoker

Adam Ainley, Rebecca Gillibrand, and Himender Makker

Case history

A 56 year old female ex-smoker was referred to a rapid access lung cancer clinic because of increasing breathlessness and weight loss. She was a healthcare professional with no past medical history except hypothyroidism. Her father had died of bowel cancer at the age of 60. On examination air entry was reduced at the right lung base. Her WHO performance status was 1. Her chest x-ray showed a right hilar mass (Fig. 10.1). A CT scan of her chest and abdomen (Fig. 10.2) was arranged prior to review in the clinic.

Questions

1. What does the CT scan of the patient's chest show?
2. What type of cancer does this patient have according to the histological and immunohistochemistry findings?
3. What samples are recommended for optimal histological evaluation?
4. Which histological features help to distinguish between different types of lung cancer?
5. Which immunohistochemical features can be used to help distinguish between types of lung cancer?
6. How would you stage this patient?

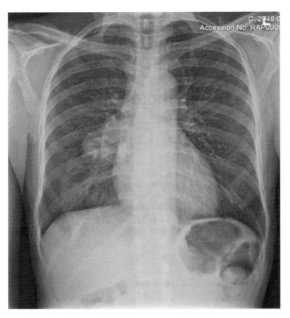

Fig. 10.1 Chest x-ray showing a right hilar mass with enlargement of the right hilum.

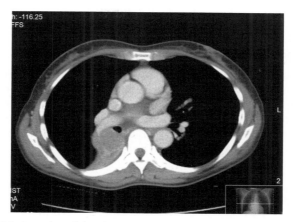

Fig. 10.2 A section of the chest CT undertaken as part of a staging scan.

Answers

1. What does the CT scan of the patient's chest show?

The CT scan shows a 3.6 cm soft tissue mass in the right hilar region with associated narrowing of the right main bronchus, right lower lobe collapse, and enlarged hilar lymph nodes. The patient also has enlarged subcarinal lymph nodes and prominent axillary and supraclavicular lymph nodes. The appearances are consistent with a primary lung malignancy with probable ipsilateral hilar lymph node and subcarinal spread but there is no evidence of distant metastasis.

Case history continued

PET-CT confirmed the findings of the staging CT. EBUS showed a friable tumour occluding the right lower lobe. On endobronchial biopsies the bronchial mucosa was infiltrated by sheets of cells with round–oval nuclei, a smooth chromatin pattern, and small amounts of cytoplasm. These cells expressed synaptophysin, focal CK7, and CD56; chromogranin, TTF-1, CK5/6, and p63 were negative. The Mib-1 monoclonal antibody labelling index revealed a high proliferation fraction.

2. What type of cancer does this patient have according to the histological and immunohistochemistry findings?

The histological appearances and IHC profile are in keeping with an SCLC. Haematoxylin and eosin (H&E) is the most useful stain for histological examination of samples in patients with suspected SCLC. It detects cells, proteins, and cell cytoplasm and is evident as a pink discoloration. Small-cell tumour cells are often small in size, less than the diameter of B lymphocytes; have round or ovoid nuclei which are often faint or absent; and have scanty cytoplasm. There is often noted to be a high mitotic rate with >70–80 mitosis/mm². Nuclear moulding is common whereas cell borders are rarely seen. IHC is often positive for neural cell adhesion molecule CD56 (90% of cases), chromogranin (60–70% of cases), and synaptophysin (60–70% of cases). Small-cell carcinomas may also express TTF-1 in 70–80% of cases. Cytokeratin AE1/AE3 is positive in the majority of cases whereas p63 is negative.

3. What samples are recommended for optimal histological evaluation?

Histological evaluation is required for confirmation of the diagnosis of lung cancer and to define the subtype. Further molecular analysis is required to determine viable therapeutic options and help predict the likely treatment response. With an increasing understanding of the underlying molecular basis of lung cancer there are now a number of targeted therapies that can be applied to particular subtypes of lung cancer; as such, obtaining a viable sample that is large enough for analysis is crucial.

When samples are not taken during direct resection it is currently recommended that both cytology and biopsy samples are obtained to increase the diagnostic yield. Cytological samples—fine needle aspirate, pleural fluid aspirate, and bronchial brushings and washings—have a good concordance with biopsy samples in differentiating NSCLC from SCLC. However, for accurate subtyping and molecular analysis a needle biopsy specimen using an 18–22 gauge needle is preferred.

Subsequent staining of samples should be undertaken using H&E, periodic acid–Schiff, and Alcian blue stains in order to optimize the pathologist's first assessment of samples, upon which a provisional diagnosis can often be made. However, given the need for subsequent molecular analysis, caution should be taken to ensure that sufficient material is left after staining for this purpose.

4. Which histological features help to distinguish between different types of lung cancer?

Previously histological typing and subtyping of lung cancer was based upon analysis of large resected samples. However, with the increasing availability of a number of less invasive sampling methods, the diagnosis of lung cancer and subtype is made on small biopsy and cytological samples. In order to reflect the greater need to define not only resected whole tumour samples but also small biopsies a number of classifications have been recommended by national and international organizations: IASLC, American and European thoracic societies, and the WHO. Lung tumours are classified into eight groups, with the main groups including adenocarcinomas, squamous cell carcinoma, and neuroendocrine tumours, which include SCLC and large-cell lung carcinoma. Less common types include adenosquamous carcinoma, sarcomatoid carcinomas, salivary gland tumours, and other/unclassified carcinomas. Within each group there are further subtypes based upon specific histological findings.

Adenocarcinomas are subclassified into five types and are broadly determined by the degree of invasion noted on resected samples, e.g. minimally invasive adenocarcinoma (in which the tumour is ≤3 cm and has ≤5 mm of an invasive component) or invasive adenocarcinoma (in which there is a >5 mm invasive component). These are then further divided according to whether or not they are mucus producing and the degree of glandular differentiation, with tumours being classified according to the predominant histological pattern including lepidic, acinar, papillary, micropapillary, or solid phase tumours.

Squamous cell carcinomas are differentiated by the degree of keratin production (keratinizing or non-keratinizing), presence of intercellular bridges and squamous pearl formation, and whether or not there is a basaloid architecture.

Large-cell lung carcinomas are predominantly those that were previously thought to be undifferentiated and are now defined as either solid adenocarcinomas or non-keratinizing squamous cell carcinoma. Diagnosis is dependent upon the presence of positive IHC results that are concordant with the underlying cell type. This group can only be defined after resection.

Neuroendocrine tumours include SCLCs, carcinoid, and other neuroendocrine tumours. SCLCs show features as discussed above. Although classified together, carcinoid tumours can be distinguished from the other types by the lower rate of mitosis and necrosis in combination with different clinical and epidemiological features.

Sarcomatoid carcinomas are very rare but are indicated when pleomorphic, epithelial spindle, or giant cells are present in 10% of the tumour biopsied.

5. Which immunohistochemical features can be used to help distinguish between types of lung cancer?

IHC is useful for both subtyping tumours and receptor typing. IHC analysis helps to identify the expression of tumour-associated antigens, such as TTF-1, CK5, CK6, CK7, and tumour protein p63, and neuroendocrine markers, such as synaptophysin, chromogranin, and nuclear adhesion molecule CD56, which can help further subtype tumours.

Adenocarcinomas are most commonly associated with the expression of TTF-1 and CK7. Squamous cell tumours are most commonly associated with the expression of CK5, CK6, and p63. Small-cell and neuroendocrine tumours are most commonly associated with expression of CD56, synaptophysin, and chromogranin.

6. How would you stage this patient?

The patient would be staged as having limited stage SCLC, T2aN2M0, on the basis of a 3.6 cm soft tissue mass, involvement of the ipsilateral hilar and subcarinal lymph nodes, but no distant metastatic disease.

Follow-up and outcome

The patient was given two cycles of chemotherapy with etoposide and carboplatin. She developed constipation and lower abdominal pain. CT scan demonstrated a new 3 cm hyperdense lesion abutting the anal canal and small bilateral inguinal lymph nodes. PET-CT and MRI followed by lymph node biopsy showed that the histology and immunoprofile were the same as the primary lung cancer and her disease had progressed to extensive stage SCLC. She received palliative radiotherapy to the anal metastases. The patient died 14 months after her initial diagnosis.

Further reading

Davidson MR, Gazdar AF, Clarke BE. The pivotal role of pathology in the management of lung cancer. J Thorac Dis. 2013 Oct;**5**(Suppl 5):S463–78.

Dietel M et al. Diagnostic procedures for non-small-cell lung cancer (NSCLC): recommendations of the European Expert Group. Thorax. 2016 Feb;**71**(2):177–84.

Dooms C, Muylle I, Yserbyt J, Ninane V. Endobronchial ultrasound in the management of non-small cell lung cancer. Eur Respir Rev. 2013 Jun;**22**(128):169–77.

Goldstein NS, Hewitt SM, Taylor CR, Yaziji H, Hicks DG; Members of Ad-Hoc Committee On Immunohistochemistry Standardization. Recommendations for improved standardization of immunohistochemistry. Appl Immunohistochem Mol Morphol. 2007 Jun;**15**(2):124–33.

Kini SR. Color Atlas of Pulmonary Cytopathology. New York, NY: Springer Verlag; 2002. pp. 3–5.

Laing GM, Chapman AD, Smart LM, Kerr KM. Histological diagnosis: recent developments. ERS Monogr. 2015;**68**:64–78.

Travis WD. Pathology of lung cancer. Clin Chest Med. 2011(32):669–92.

Travis WD. Update on small cell carcinoma and its differentiation from squamous cell carcinoma and other non-small cell carcinomas. Mod Pathol. 2012 Jan;**25**(Suppl 1):S18–30.

Travis WD et al. International Association for the Study of Lung Cancer/American Thoracic Society/European Respiratory Society international multidisciplinary classification of lung adenocarcinoma. J Thorac Oncol 2011;**6**(2):244–85.

Travis WD et al. The 2015 World Health Organization classification of lung tumours. Impact of genetic, clinical and radiological advances since the 2004 classification. J Thorac Oncol. 2015 Sep;**10**(9):1243–60.

Wu CC et al. CT-guided percutaneous needle biopsy of the chest: pre-procedural evaluation and technique. AJR Am J Roentgenol. 2011;**196**:W511–14.

Case 11

Pericardial and pleural effusions in a smoker with metastatic adenocarcinoma

Adam Ainley, Rebecca Gillibrand, and Himender Makker

Case history

A 54 year old female smoker of 15 pack-years was referred by her GP to a cardiologist because of right-sided chest pain, exertional breathlessness, and cardiac enlargement on chest x-ray. Further investigation revealed a pericardial effusion, and pericardiocentesis was performed. The fluid obtained contained no evidence of infection, and no malignant cells were identified on microscopy.

CT scan revealed changes consistent with metastatic cancer. A right hilar mass was present with right hilar lymphadenopathy, right lower lobe collapse, and right pleural effusion. The pericardium was thickened and irregular. Lytic lesions were noted in the T3 vertebral body and multiple hypodense lesions were present in the liver.

A pleural aspirate of yellow fluid was obtained. Cytological (ThinPrep) and cell block examination revealed a moderately cellular sample containing small papillary clusters of atypical epithelioid cells with pleomorphic nuclei, prominent nucleoli, and vacuolated cytoplasm in a background of benign mesothelial cells, mixed inflammatory cells, and blood. Their immunocytochemical profile was: CK7 positive, TTF-1 positive, CEA positive, ER negative, WT-1 negative, and CK20 negative.

Her case was discussed at the lung MDT meeting and liver biopsy was recommended for histological confirmation.

Questions

1. What is the most likely type of lung malignancy associated with these cytological and immunocytochemical findings?
2. Which additional tests would help in guiding this patient's treatment options?
3. What are the indications for mutation analysis?
4. What does mutation analysis detect?
5. What type of samples can be sent for molecular analysis?

Answers

1. What is the most likely type of lung malignancy associated with these cytological and immunocytochemical findings?

Adenocarcinoma is the most likely malignancy. Adenocarcinoma is an epithelial malignancy which often forms papillary clusters in cytological preparations. The combination of CK7 and TTF-1 is commonly expressed in adenocarcinoma of primary lung origin. CEA is expressed by many adenocarcinomas, including those arising from the lung and the gastrointestinal tract. ER may be expressed by adenocarcinomas from the breast or female genital tract. WT-1 may be expressed by epithelial tumours of ovarian and fallopian tube origin, and by mesothelioma. CK20 is often expressed by adenocarcinomas of lower gastrointestinal tract origin.

The liver biopsy showed liver tissue infiltrated by moderately differentiated adenocarcinoma. IHC demonstrated tumour cells expressing CK7 and TTF-1. ER, PgR, and CK20 were negative. The appearances and IHC support a primary lung origin.

2. Which additional tests would help in guiding this patient's treatment options?

Greater understanding of the underlying molecular basis of lung cancers has allowed the development of targeted therapies towards specific tumour types based upon their associated genetic abnormalities. The most commonly targeted abnormalities are associated with NSCLC and include EGFR mutations and rearrangements of the ALK gene. In the UK 16.6% of patients with NSCLC have been found to be EGFR mutation positive whereas 3–5% of patients have the ALK gene rearrangement. Other less commonly used molecular biomarkers and therapeutic targets undergoing further evaluation include v-RAF murine sarcoma viral oncogene homologue B (BRAF), human epidermal growth factor receptor (HER), Kirsten rat sarcoma viral oncogene homologue (KRAS), and ROS proto-oncogene 1 receptor tyrosine kinase (ROS-1).

EGFR mutations and ALK rearrangements provide therapeutic targets for TKIs such as erlotinib and crizotinib and provide additional treatment options for patients with newly diagnosed or recurrent NSCLC or for those who did not respond to first-line therapy.

Case history continued

Analysis for EGFR mutation demonstrated a point mutation p.L858R in exon 21, thus there was an increased likelihood of response to TKI treatment.

3. What are the indications for mutation analysis?

It is currently recommended that EGFR and ALK mutation analysis be undertaken in all patients presenting with:

1. locally advanced or metastatic lung adenocarcinoma
2. recurrence of adenocarcinoma
3. failure of response to first-line therapy or EGFR/ALK-targeted therapies.

4. What does mutation analysis detect?

Mutation analysis for EGFR detects the most commonly found mutations associated with NSCLC, which include a deletion in exon 19 and a point mutation in exon 21, L858R. Mutation analysis is undertaken using DNA extracted from biopsy samples. ALK mutations can be identified using IHC-related antibodies, with fluorescence *in situ* hybridization or using polymerase chain reaction-based methods.

5. What type of samples can be sent for molecular analysis?

Tissue specimens remain the gold standard for any molecular assays; however, cytological samples can be used when no other samples are available. Molecular analysis requires a highly cellular sample to increase its sensitivity. Cytological specimens have been shown to have comparable sensitivity to biopsy samples in some studies.

Follow-up and outcome

The patient was diagnosed with stage IV T1–2NxM1b adenocarcinoma of the lung and commenced on palliative chemotherapy with cisplatin and pemetrexed while awaiting the results of the mutation analysis. She did not tolerate the first cycle well. She was treated with erlotinib in view of her EGFR-positive status and remained clinically stable for a year.

Further reading

Cree IA et al. Guidance for laboratories performing molecular pathology for cancer patients. J Clin Pathol. 2014 Nov;**67**(11):923–31.

Dietel M et al. Diagnostic procedures for non-small-cell lung cancer (NSCLC): recommendations of the European Expert Group. Thorax. 2016 Feb;**71**(2):177–84.

Kim L, Tsao MS. Tumour tissue sampling for lung cancer management in the era of personalised therapy: what is good enough for molecular testing? Eur Respir J. 2014 Oct;**44**(4):1011–22.

Lindeman NI et al. Molecular testing guideline for selection of patients for EGFR and ALK tyrosine kinase inhibitors: guideline from the College of American Pathologists, International Association for the Study of Lung Cancer and Association for Molecular Pathology. J Thorac Oncol. 2013 Jul;**8**(7):823–59.

Nana-Sinkam SP et al. Molecular Biology of Lung Cancer: Diagnosis and Management of Lung Cancer 3rd ed: ACCP guidelines. Chest. 2013: **143**(5 Suppl):e30S–e39S.

National Institute for Health and Care Excellence. EGFR-TK Mutation Testing in Adults with Locally Advanced or Metastatic Non-Small Cell Lung Cancer. Diagnostics Guidance DG9. London, UK: NICE; 2013.

Wood SL, Pernemalm M, Crosbie PA, Whetton AD. Molecular histology of lung cancer: from targets to treatments. Cancer Treat Rev. 2015 Apr;**41** (4):361–75.

Case 12

Right lower lobe squamous cell carcinoma associated with hilar and mediastinal lymphadenopathy

Adam Ainley, Bryan Sheinman,
and Himender Makker

Case history

A 60 year old Turkish female was referred to a rapid access respiratory clinic with a 6 month history of weight loss, reduced appetite, breathlessness on moderate exertion, intermittent cough with white sputum, and slight hoarseness of voice. She was a tobacco smoker with a 40 pack-year history. Her father died of lung cancer in his sixties. On examination there was a 1 cm, palpable nodule in the right anterior triangle of the neck. Respiratory and general examinations were otherwise unremarkable and WHO performance status was 1. A CT chest scan (Fig. 12.1) revealed a 1 × 2.6 cm peripheral, posterior, right lower lobe mass abutting the chest wall. A 1.5 cm short-axis diameter subcarinal node was noted, but no other nodes were enlarged by CT criteria.

Questions

1. How do you classify an enlarged pulmonary lymph node?

2. What investigations would you request at this stage?

3. What is the provisional radiological staging and how would you investigate this patient further?

4. How is lymph node involvement classified according to TNM criteria?

5. What other investigations can be used for staging of lymph node involvement and mediastinal staging?

6. What are the recommended indications for mediastinal histological staging?

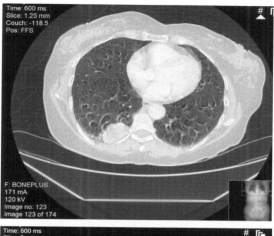

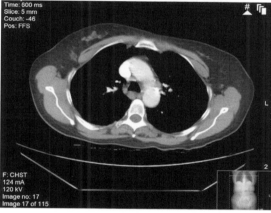

Fig. 12.1 CT chest scan showing a right lower lobe mass and subcarinal lymphadenopathy.

Answers

1. How do you classify an enlarged pulmonary lymph node?

Lymph nodes are enlarged by CT Criteria when they are >10 mm in the short-axis diameter. Nodes of <10 mm are considered within normal limits, those of 10–20 mm are referred to as 'small volume' lymph nodes, and those >20 mm in the short-axis diameter are classified as 'bulky'.

Lymph node enlargement is further stratified according to the likely probability of associated mediastinal malignancy, with those <10 mm being considered to be of low probability (15%), those between 10 and 20 mm of intermediate probability (50%), and those >20 mm of high probability (85%) of mediastinal malignancy. Enlarged lymph nodes with heterogeneous echogenicity on US or loss of the normal fatty central region on CT are more likely to be malignant. FDG-avid lymph nodes on PET scan have a high probability of mediastinal malignancy.

Case history continued

The patient had a 1.5 cm subcarinal node enlargement and a further sample was required to exclude mediastinal involvement.

2. What investigations would you request at this stage?

A finding of a 1 cm neck mass is suggestive of an enlarged anterior cervical lymph node.

In patients with N3 disease including low cervical, supraclavicular, or sternal notch lymphadenopathy on physical examination and/or on CT or PET-CT, histological confirmation with a US-guided FNA biopsy is recommended. Histological confirmation of extrathoracic N3 nodal disease avoids the need for mediastinal staging.

Case history continued

US of the neck was performed and showed a cyst that was likely to be sebaceous in origin, thus ruling out N3 disease. PET-CT was requested to characterize the underlying abnormalities and to look for evidence of further nodal disease and/or distant metastasis. It revealed a peripheral posteriorly placed 4.4 × 3.0 cm mass in the right lower lobe with intense FDG uptake (SUV_{max} = 22.5). The mass extended posteriorly but there was no convincing evidence of rib, pleura, or chest wall involvement. No other FDG-avid lung nodules were noted. Mildly FDG-avid right hilar (SUV_{max} = 2.8), subcarinal (SUV_{max} = 2.5), prevascular, right paratracheal, and anterior–superior mediastinal nodes were noted. There was no FDG-avid disease below the diaphragm. A 1 cm, well-defined, non-FDG-avid, low-density lesion in the subcutaneous tissue at the level of the right mandibular angle was deemed likely to represent a cyst. In summary, the PET-CT demonstrated an FDG-avid, right lower lobe lung mass with mediastinal nodal disease.

3. What is the provisional radiological staging and how would you investigate this patient further?

The CT and PET-CT findings suggest a stage of T2aN2M0, depending upon further mediastinal staging.

Case history continued

The MDT recommended CT-guided biopsy of the right lower lobe lesion and EBUS-TBNA for assessment of mediastinal node involvement.

4. How is lymph node involvement classified according to TNM criteria?

Lymph node disease is divided into five categories (Nx and N0–N3) according to the seventh edition of the TNM criteria and is depicted in a lymph node map proposed by the IASLC and the American Joint Committee on Cancer.

Nx denotes when no sampling can be undertaken of regional lymph nodes.

N0 denotes no evidence of lymph node metastasis.

N1 involvement refers to lymph node involvement in the ipsilateral peribronchial (i.e. paratracheal) and/or ipsilateral hilar and/or intrapulmonary nodes. These are also referred to as stations 10 (hilar), 11 (interlobar), 12 (lobar), 13 (segmental), and 14 (subsegmental).

N2 disease refers to the involvement of subcarinal lymph nodes (also known as station 7), with or without ipsilateral nodal involvement.

N3 disease refers to involvement of the contralateral mediastinal or hilar nodes or any scalene or supraclavicular lymph nodes (station 1).

5. What other investigations can be used for staging of lymph node involvement and mediastinal staging?

Mediastinal and lymph nodes can be sampled either with EBUS-TBNA or with endoscopic ultrasound (EUS)-guided FNA via the oesophagus. These techniques are able to visualize lymph nodes ≥5 mm and can be used in combination. EBUS-accessible stations include some N1 (although nodes distal to the hilum may be difficult or impossible to sample), inferior mediastinal nodes (N2, station 7), and the superior mediastinal nodes at stations 2, 3p, and 4. All FDG-positive nodes or the largest node in each station should be biopsied. Biopsies should be taken from the most distal station first to avoid contamination of samples, and three samples should be taken during the procedure to ensure an adequate amount of material for subsequent analysis if rapid on-site evaluation (ROSE) is not available (ROSE refers to immediate histological examination of samples at the time of the procedure but is not practical in all centres). EUS can be used to sample stations 4L, 7, 8, and 9. Samples can also be taken from the left adrenal gland and the left lobe of the liver using EUS (but not EBUS), whereas EBUS-TBNA can be used to sample stations 2, 4, 7, and 10 (+/−11).

When endoscopic methods are unsuccessful and malignancy is still suspected, surgical options include mediastinoscopy to sample stations 1, 2–4, 7, and 10 or VATS, which can also be used to sample stations 5 and 6 (para- and subaortic), which are inaccessible by other methods, as well as stations 7, 8, and 9. VATS also allows direct sampling of single or multiple peripheral pulmonary lesions.

6. What are the recommended indications for mediastinal histological staging?

Mediastinal histological staging prior to initiation of therapy is indicated in:

1. Patients with NSCLC who are deemed suitable for radical (surgical) intervention/treatments with curative intent.
2. Patients with lymph node enlargement of 10 mm short-axis diameter on CT- or PET-CT-positive ipsilateral hilar nodes.
3. A suspected primary tumour despite low FDG avidity on PET-CT.

Mediastinal histological staging is not indicated in patients with peripheral lesions of <3 cm without evidence of mediastinal or hilar lymph node enlargement or positivity on CT/PET-CT.

Follow-up and outcome

CT-guided biopsy showed cores of lung tissue infiltrated by poorly differentiated NSCLC, with cells expressing AE1/AE3, CK5/6, and p63. Some of the tumour cells did show TTF-1 positivity but CK7 was negative. These morphological and immunohistochemical features are in keeping with squamous cell carcinoma. EBUS-TBNA was undertaken at stations 7 and 4R with good quality samples and no malignant cells were seen. Final staging was T2aN0M0, stage IB with good performance status, and right lower lobectomy was performed with curative intent.

Further reading

Dooms C, Decaluwe H, De Leyn P. Mediastinal staging. Eur Respir Monogr. 2015;**68**:159–66.

El-Sherief AH, Lau CT, Wu CC, Drake RL, Abbott GF, Rice TW. International Association for the Study of Lung Cancer (IASLC) lymph node map: radiologic review with CT illustration. RadioGraphics. 2014;**34**(6):1680–91.

Lim E et al. Guidelines on the radical management of patients with lung cancer. Thorax. 2010;**65**(Suppl III):iii1–iii27.

Padhani AR. Lymph nodes. In: Nicholson T, editor. Recommendations for Cross Sectional Imaging in Cancer Management. Second edition. London, UK: Royal College of Radiologists; 2014.

Rusch VW et al. The IASLC lung cancer staging project: a proposal for a new international lymph node map in the forthcoming seventh edition of the TNM classification for lung cancer. J Thorac Oncol. 2009;**4**(5):568–77.

Terán MD, Broch MV. Staging of lymph node metastases from lung cancer in the mediastinum. J Thorac Dis. 2014;**6**(3)230–6.

Travis WD et al. International Association for the Study of Lung Cancer/American Thoracic Society/European Respiratory Society international multidisciplinary classification of lung adenocarcinoma. J Thorac Oncol. 2011;**6**(2):244–85.

Vilmann P et al. Combined endobronchial and oesophageal endosonography for diagnosis and staging of lung cancer. European Society of Gastrointestinal Endoscopy (ESGE) guideline, in cooperation with the European Respiratory Society (ERS) and the European Society of Thoracic Surgeons (ESTS). Eur Respir J. 2015 Jul;**46**(1):40–60.

Case 13

A 30 year old female with a solitary lesion and haemoptysis

Adam Ainley and Himender Makker

Case history

A 30 year old female of African origin who had never smoked was referred to the lung cancer clinic having presented to her GP with a 2 month history of recurrent cough and haemoptysis. At onset this was a dry cough associated with fever and nasal discharge. She subsequently developed right-sided chest pains. Despite two courses of antibiotics her symptoms did not resolve. Her exercise tolerance was stable but she felt fatigued; she denied any breathlessness. She was previously diagnosed with asthma but had no other relevant medical history other than an aunt who had a form of cancer, site unknown to her. Clinical examination was unremarkable. Her WHO performance status was 0 and lung function revealed normal spirometry and gas transfer.

A chest x-ray undertaken prior to her review in the clinic is shown in Fig. 13.1.

Questions

1. What does the chest x-ray show?
2. What is the role of CT in the initial investigation of patients with suspected lung cancer?
3. What other imaging modalities have a role in the initial evaluation of patients with suspected lung cancer?
4. Is there a role for PET-CT imaging in the management of this patient?
5. What type of tumour are the patient's histological findings consistent with?

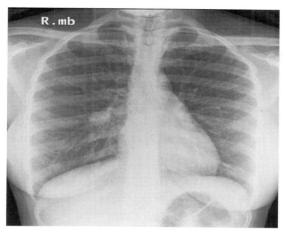

Fig. 13.1 Abnormal chest x-ray.

Answers

1. What does the chest x-ray show?

There is a well-defined right-sided hilar opacity.

An urgent chest x-ray should be requested for all patients presenting with persistent symptoms/signs lasting more than 3 weeks that are suggestive of underlying malignancy. These include cough, chest/shoulder pain, breathlessness, weight or appetite loss, haemoptysis, and palpable lymphadenopathy, e.g. cervical/supraclavicular.

All patients with worrying chest x-ray findings or symptoms should be referred urgently to the lung cancer MDT; in most cases this is likely to be via a local respiratory consultant. The referral should be guided by an underlying clinical suspicion even if the initial chest x-ray is reported as normal. Referral should be expedited if there are any underlying signs of superior vena cava obstruction, severe airway obstruction, e.g. stridor, or persistent haemoptysis in any patient aged over 40 years irrespective of smoking status.

Case history continued

In light of the patient's history, upon triaging the referrals, the local respiratory consultant arranged for an urgent CT scan of her chest to be undertaken prior to the patient's attendance in the clinic; the results are shown in Fig. 13.2.

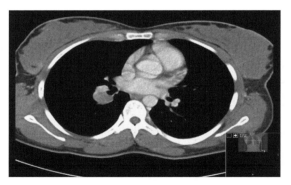

Fig. 13.2 CT chest demonstrates a 2 × 2 cm smooth enhancing mass lesion at the lower pole of the right hilum. Enhancement was up to 94 Hounsfield units. No associated fat or calcification noted.

2. What is the role of CT in the initial investigation of patients with suspected lung cancer?

Contrast-enhanced CT of both the chest and abdomen is recommended in all patients with suspected lung cancer in order to characterize any focal lesions and the extent of any associated nodal or metastatic involvement. Early use of CT in the clinical evaluation of patients with suspected lung cancer facilitates the appropriate selection of diagnostic tests and allows provisional staging of any disease. CT has an overall sensitivity of 89–100% but a low specificity of 56–63% for lung cancer, and a lower sensitivity at approximately 55% for staging of nodal disease. CT primarily has a role in identifying any enlarged lymph nodes and providing information on their likely site. This information is useful in guiding further imaging and procedures aimed at obtaining histological and cytological confirmation. Because of the lack of specificity histological confirmation should always be sought to confirm/exclude malignancy in any lesions or any enlarged lymph nodes seen. CT is, however, used in the staging of SCLC, in which it is considered reliable at differentiating between limited and extensive disease.

It is recommended that a CT chest scan should be undertaken prior to any interventional procedures to ensure optimal localization of target lesions and guide the site of biopsies.

Case history continued

In light of the patient's CT findings an FB was performed to evaluate the primary lesion, and further imaging was requested to exclude any nodal or metastatic disease.

3. What other imaging modalities have a role in the initial evaluation of patients with suspected lung cancer?

Although CT is useful in helping to identify any lesions and highlight any lymph node involvement, it is less reliable when evaluating lesions that invade adjacent structures such as the chest wall, pleura, local vessels, and other structures.

MRI has been shown to be more reliable than contrast-enhanced CT in the assessment of chest wall invasion. Furthermore, MRI is the most efficient modality for assessing apical/superior lung lesions and is frequently used in the diagnosis of Pancoast tumours. Although MRI has been advocated for use in the evaluation of chest wall lesions and Pancoast tumours, it has a much lower range of sensitivity (90–96%) and specificity (57–100%) for staging of NSCLC than PET-CT.

US is not viable as a staging modality and is not routinely recommended in this role. There is, however, a role for US in guiding percutaneous needle biopsy of distant metastatic lesions, such as liver, adrenal, and pleural lesions, or abnormal lymph nodes seen on other staging scans. US is particularly useful in staging supraclavicular node involvement/N3 disease.

4. Is there a role for PET-CT imaging in the management of this patient?

This patient has a WHO performance status of 0. Taking this into account with her lung function and CT findings of a solitary left upper lobe lesion she would be a viable candidate for radical/curative intervention. In all patients with suspected lung cancer deemed suitable for radical interventions a PET/PET-CT is recommended.

PET-CT is recommended as the next radiological investigation after conventional CT of the thorax and abdomen in order to assess for evidence of regional lymph node involvement and to detect distant metastases.

PET-CT is useful to assess mediastinal disease when CT has demonstrated mediastinal lymph node enlargement described as either high probability of mediastinal malignancy (defined as lymph nodes >20 mm maximum short-axis diameter) or intermediate probability of mediastinal malignancy (defined as lymph nodes of 10–20 mm short-axis diameter). Meta-analysis of relevant studies has demonstrated that PET-CT has a false negative rate of around 5% for mediastinal lymph nodes of <10 mm on short-axis diameter compared with 21% for nodes >15 mm. Therefore, patients should proceed to radical treatment if mediastinal nodes on CT are <10 mm and the PET-CT is negative. Sampling is needed for all mediastinal nodes if they are >10 mm on CT or are positive on PET.

Case history continued

Following the contrast-enhanced CT the patient underwent PET-CT to assess for mediastinal disease and distant metastases. This revealed a low-grade uptake of SUV_{max} = 3.5. The possibility of an underlying carcinoid lesion was suggested and subsequently a whole-body Ga-DOTATATE (octreotide) scan was undertake but demonstrated a very low uptake of 1 within the lesion, as shown in Figs 13.3 and 13.4.

In light of her clinical symptoms and radiological investigations a bronchoscopy and EBUS were undertaken. No obvious endobronchial component was seen but EBUS-TBNA demonstrated sheets of polygonal bland cells with central ovoid nuclei and eosinophilic granular cytoplasm. IHC showed cytoplasmic positivity for S100 and negative results for cytokeratin AE1–3 and CD163.

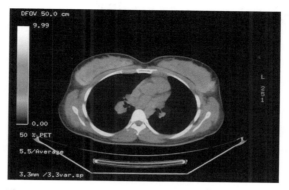

Fig. 13.3 Whole-body Ga-DOTATATE (octreotide).

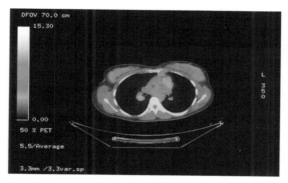

Fig. 13.4 PET-CT.

5. What type of tumour are the patient's histological findings consistent with?

The histological and morphological features of the patient's tumour are consistent with a diagnosis of a benign granular cell tumour (GCT). This is thought to arise from Schwann cells, and is a rare tumour type first described in 1926 by Abrikossoff in a case series of tongue-associated tumours. The first case associated within the endobronchial tree was documented in the 1930s. Endobronchial cases remain rare at fewer than 100 worldwide, with most cases reported in various other body sites, including subcutaneous tissue, breast, skin, oral cavity, and abdominal wall. Of the cases reported 6% are in the tracheobronchial tree and GCTs constitute only 0.2% of all pulmonary cancers.

Most GCTs are slow growing; however, malignant change has been noted with regional lymphatic spread and distant metastasis. Treatment options are not clearly defined given the rarity of the tumour type, although most commonly they involve curative surgical resection, either segmental or lobar, especially when there is associated obstruction of the bronchial tree. Other options include endoscopic resection, cryotherapy, and laser photocoagulation.

Follow-up and outcome

After further discussion at the lung cancer MDT meeting the patient was deemed suitable for surgical intervention and was referred to the thoracic surgeons. She consented to undergo a VATS lobectomy, which was undertaken and was thought curative. She has been well since with ongoing follow-up.

Further reading

Hernandez OG, Hapnoik EF, Summer WR. Granular cell tumour of the bronchus: bronchoscopic and clinical features. Thorax. 1986 Dec;41(12):927–31.

Monnier-Cholley L, Arrivé L, Porcel A, Shehata K, Dahan H, Urban T, Febvre M, Lebeau B, Tubiana JM. Characteristics of missed lung cancer on chest radiographs: a French experience. Eur Radiol. 2001;11(4):597–605.

National Institute for Health and Care Excellence. Lung Cancer: Diagnosis and Management. Clinical Guideline 121. London, UK: NICE; 2011. pp. 32–43.

Quekel LG, Kessels AG, Goei R, van Engelshoven JM. Miss rate of lung cancer on the chest radiograph in clinical practice. Chest. 1999 Mar;115(3):720–4.

Scottish Intercollegiate Guidelines Network. Management of Lung Cancer. SIGN publication no. 137. Edinburgh, UK: SIGN; 2014. pp. 13–20.

Silvestri GA, Gonzalez AV, Jantz MA, Margolis ML, Gould MK, Tanoue LT, Harris LJ, Detterbeck FC. Methods for staging non-small cell lung cancer: diagnosis and management of lung cancer, 3rd ed: American College of Chest Physicians evidence-based clinical practice guidelines, Chest. 2013;143(Suppl 5):e211s–e250s.

Case 14

Asymptomatic metastatic disease in a 71 year old male with a history of frequent falls

Adam Ainley and Himender Makker

Case history

A 71 year old male was referred to a rapid access lung cancer clinic having attended an accident and emergency department due to recurrent falls. As part of his assessment he was found to have an abnormal chest x-ray (Fig. 14.1). On further review he denied any respiratory symptoms and had no constitutional symptoms. He had had a number of falls over the last few years that had been attributed to frailty, for which he received physiotherapy and occupational therapy. His wife also reported concerns regarding his memory and he was due to attend a memory clinic. His past medical history included depression, hypothyroidism, hypertension, type 2 diabetes mellitus, previous transient ischaemic attack, and hypercholesterolaemia. He was an ex-tobacco smoker with a 30 pack-year history. His current medications included clopidogrel as well as antihypertensive and oral diabetic therapy. Further physical examination was unremarkable. He had an abbreviated mental test score of 8/10 and his WHO performance status was between 2 and 3. A contrast-enhanced staging CT of his chest and abdomen was subsequently requested (Fig. 14.2).

Questions

1. What does the patient's chest x-ray show?

2. What does the patient's CT scan show?

3. What further investigations would you request on the basis of the patient's clinical history, performance status, and radiological investigations?

4. What is the frequency and significance of metastatic disease in the diagnosis of lung cancer?

5. What options are available for further investigation of underlying distant extrathoracic (M1b) metastatic disease?

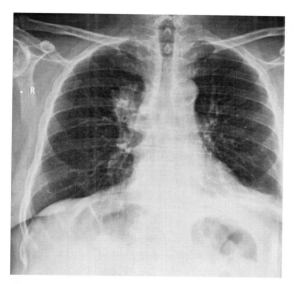

Fig. 14.1 Chest x-ray.

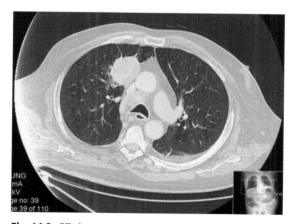

Fig. 14.2 CT chest.

Answers

1. What does the patient's chest x-ray show?

The patient's chest x-ray demonstrates a right upper lobe mass adjacent to the right hilum that warrants further investigation with a staging CT.

2. What does the patient's CT scan show?

The CT scan shows an approximately 4 cm soft tissue mass in the right upper chest, adjacent to the mediastinum and associated with mediastinal lymphadenopathy. Some consolidation is also visible at the left base with a small effusion.

Case history continued

A 2 × 1.5 cm nodule can be seen in the right adrenal gland with a further 3.5 cm nodule involving the inferior aspect of the left adrenal gland.

3. What further investigations would you request on the basis of the patient's clinical history, performance status, and radiological investigations?

The primary concern is that this patient has an underlying malignancy with evidence of mediastinal involvement and distant metastasis. As such it would be prudent to seek a histological confirmation of the diagnosis. However, in light of his multiple comorbidities and less than optimal performance status a less invasive option such as a transthoracic image-guided biopsy would be considered the most optimal choice.

Case history continued

His case was discussed at the lung MDT meeting and in light of his relative frailty it was felt appropriate to undertake a CT-guided biopsy rather than a more invasive approach (Fig. 14.3) in order to obtain a histological diagnosis.

The patient's CT-guided biopsy demonstrated cores of lung tissue infiltrated by NSCLC with IHC revealing tumour cells expressing CK7 and TTF-1. CK5/6, p63, and CK20 were negative. The morphological features favoured adenocarcinoma, which was supported by the immunoprofile and was in keeping with a primary lung origin.

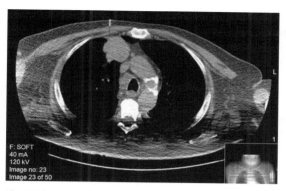

Fig. 14.3 CT-guided biopsy.

4. What is the frequency and significance of metastatic disease in the diagnosis of lung cancer?

Metastatic disease is common in patients presenting with lung carcinoma. Up to 40% of patients with NSCLC and over 60% of patients with SCLC present with advanced disease and metastasis. The most common sites of metastatic disease in order of frequency include: the brain (15–43%), liver (33–40%), bone (19–33%), adrenal glands (18–38%), kidney (16–23%), and lung (10–15%), with metastasis also seen to a lower frequency in the pancreas, in the spleen, and subcutaneously. Approximately 10% of patients, such as this patient, present with asymptomatic metastatic disease.

Optimal assessment for, and the exclusion of, metastatic disease is an important step in the evaluation of patients presenting with suspected lung cancer. Metastatic disease confirms stage IV disease. It is recommended that metastatic disease for all types of cancers is defined on the basis of the seventh edition of the TNM classification. Historically, the extent of SCLC disease was classified into two stages—either limited or extensive disease—using the VALG criteria; although still mentioned, these criteria have been superseded by the TNM criteria.

Staging of metastatic disease is divided into either thoracic (M1a) or extrathoracic (M1b) involvement. M1a lesions include those within the contralateral lung, pulmonary nodules within the same lung associated with the primary lesion, or an associated malignant pericardial or pleural effusion. M1b lesions are any that are extrathoracic, including bone, liver, adrenal, and cerebral metastases.

5. What options are available for further investigation of underlying distant extrathoracic (M1b) metastatic disease?

Thoracic metastatic disease is investigated in a similar fashion to primary lesions and has been discussed in earlier sections. Investigation of extrathoracic metastatic lung disease is mainly recommended for patients in whom curative or intensive treatment options are being considered. Focused imaging should be guided by clinical evaluation. PET-CT is the initial radiological investigation undertaken to exclude distant metastatic disease.

Assessment of brain metastases. Brain metastases are a common occurrence in patients with lung carcinoma. Contrast-enhanced CT and/or MRI of the brain is recommended in patients with symptoms suggestive of underlying lesions or in those who are asymptomatic but have disease elsewhere that is considered suitable for intensive/curative treatment, e.g. stage III or N2 stage disease or less. PET-CT is not reliable because of the high metabolism of glucose within cerebral structures, which makes the study difficult to interpret. There is no current recommended guideline on the sampling of brain metastasis and this is not routinely undertaken.

Liver and adrenal metastases. Both liver and adrenal metastases are common in patients with lung carcinoma; however, steps must be taken to ensure that any lesions seen on radiological investigations are not benign, given the implications for subsequent decision-making. Benign liver and adrenal lesions are common and therefore further assessment is required. It is recommended that liver lesions of >10 mm on CT require further assessment and FDG PET-CT is one modality used to investigate these, along with MRI and US. Equally PET-CT has been demonstrated to detect adrenal lesions with a sensitivity of 94–100% and a specificity of 80–100%. However, meta-analysis has demonstrated both a false negative and false positive rate of around 5% for PET-CT in assessing adrenal metastases; as such, although a negative FDG PET-CT can reliably exclude adrenal disease, when scans are thought to be indeterminate further assessment is recommended via adrenal-specific CT or MRI. When underlying malignant adrenal or liver abnormalities are suspected, further sampling by percutaneous needle biopsy is recommended for definitive confirmation. Image-guided (US or CT) percutaneous needle biopsy is thought to be accurate in 90% of cases. Although considered a safe procedure overall, the major complication is bleeding.

Bone metastasis. FDG PET-CT has been demonstrated to be more specific and sensitive than isotope bone scans. If positive for bone metastases, it can negate the need for further investigation unless cord compression is suspected. When a PET-CT is not recommended or required, a ^{99m}Tc nuclear bone scan is a viable alternative. However, current recommendations suggest additional confirmatory investigations such as focal x-rays and MRI. MRI should be the first investigation when there is concern regarding spinal cord involvement.

Follow-up and outcome

After further discussion at the MDT meeting this patient was deemed to have a poor functional baseline as he had deteriorated physically since his initial presentation with a WHO performance status of 3. In light of this, further imaging such as PET-CT or investigation of his adrenal lesion were not recommended. The decision was discussed with his family. As he remained otherwise asymptomatic, the agreed best course of action was to follow him up as required and manage any symptoms conservatively. He was supported by the local lung cancer nurses with further clinical review as required.

Further reading

Bülzebruck H, Bopp R, Drings P, Bauer E, Krysa S, Probst G, van Kaick G, Müller KM, Vogt-Moykopf I. New aspects in the staging of lung cancer. Prospective validation of the International Union Against Cancer TNM classification. Cancer. 1992 Sep;**70**(5):1102–10.

Detterbeck FC, Rivera MP, Socinski M, > Rosenman J. Diagnosis and Treatment of Lung Cancer: an Evidence-Based Guide for the Practicing Clinician. Philadelphia, PA: W.B. Saunders; 2001. p. 96.

Hillers TK, Sauve MD, Guyatt GH. Analysis of published studies on the detection of extrathoracic metastases in patients presumed to have operable non-small cell lung cancer. Thorax. 1994 Jan;**49**(1):14–19.

Kloos RT, Korobkin M, Thompson NW, Francis IR, Shapiro B, Gross MD. Incidentally discovered adrenal masses. Endocr Rev. 1995;**16**(4):460–84.

Martino CR, Haaga JR, Bryan PJ, LiPuma JP, El Yousef SJ, Alfidi RJ. CT-guided liver biopsies: eight years' experience. Work in progress. Radiology. 1984;**152**(3):755–7.

Quinn DL, Ostrow LB, Porter DK, Shelton DKJr, Jackson DEJr. Staging of non-small cell bronchogenic carcinoma. Relationship of the clinical evaluation to organ scans. Chest. 1986;**89**(2):270–5.

Quint LE, Tummala S, Brisson LJ, Francis IR, Krupnick AS, Kazerooni EA, Iannettoni MD, Whyte RI, Orringer MB. Distribution of distant metastases from newly diagnosed non-small cell lung cancer. Ann Thorac Surg. 1996 Jul;**62**(1):246–50.

Rich AL, Tata LJ, Stanley RA, Free CM, Peake MD, Baldwin DR, Hubbard RB. Lung cancer in England: information from the National Lung Cancer Audit (LUCADA). Lung Cancer. 2011 Apr;**72**(1):16–22.

Silvestri GA, Gould MK, Margolis ML, Tanoue LT, McCrory D, Toloza E, Detterbeck F; American College of Chest Physicians. Noninvasive staging of non-small cell lung cancer: ACCP evidenced-based clinical practice guidelines (2nd edition). Chest 2007 Sep;**132**(3 Suppl):178S–201S.

Walters S et al. Lung cancer survival and stage at diagnosis in Australia, Canada, Denmark, Norway, Sweden and the UK: a population-based study, 2004–2007. Thorax. 2013 Jun;**68**(6): 551–64.

Welch TJ, Sheedy PF2nd, Stephens DH, Johnson CM, Swensen SJ. Percutaneous adrenal biopsy: review of a 10-year experience. Radiology. 1994;**193**(2):341–4.

Section II

Medical oncology

Case 15

Metastatic small-cell cancer presenting with haemoptysis and left upper lobe collapse, treated with chemotherapy

Oscar Juan and Sanjay Popat

Case history

A 63 year old male presented to an accident and emergency department with a persistent cough and haemoptysis. He had a 90 pack-year smoking history, and was currently smoking two packs of cigarettes daily. He had been treated a month before with antibiotics for cough and fever. His fever disappeared and his cough improved on antibiotic therapy. He presented with a 2 day history of productive cough and haemoptysis. He was hypertensive and had had a myocardial infarction 10 years previously. His current medications included antihypertensives and aspirin. He had no known drug allergies.

The patient's physical examination findings were normal. His Eastern Cooperative Oncology Group (ECOG) performance status was 1. Chest x-ray revealed a mass in the left upper lobe associated with lobar collapse. The patient was referred to the chest team, which ordered a CT scan that confirmed the presence of a 6 × 5 cm mass in the left upper lobe that was obstructing the main left bronchus, producing atelectasis. Additionally, enlarged mediastinal nodes were observed in the left high and low paratracheal, precarinal, and subcarinal areas. The CT scan including the liver and the adrenal glands did not show any metastatic lesions. Haematology and blood chemistry did not reveal any significant findings. A bronchoscopic biopsy confirmed small-cell lung cancer (SCLC). Immunohistochemical staining with synaptophysin, pan-cytokeratin, and chromogranin was positive.

Questions

1. What further investigations would you request?
2. What stage is the patient's disease?
3. What treatment would you offer to this patient? If you would offer radiation therapy, would you administer it concurrently or sequentially?
4. What toxicities would you expect from the treatment?
5. Would you recommend any further treatment at this point?
6. What would you recommend in this situation?

Answers

1. What further investigations would you request?

In addition to a CT scan of the chest and abdomen, when the metastatic stage is not obvious bone scintigraphy or PET-CT and brain MRI are recommended for initial staging of SCLC to rule out bone and brain metastasis. Although CT scanning with intravenous contrast of the brain is an alternative, MRI is preferred because of its greater sensitivity in detecting brain metastases. Instead of a CT scan and bone scintigraphy, staging can be performed with a fludeoxyglucose (FDG) PET-CT scan. PET-CT is superior to other radiological methods at identifying latent sites of metastatic disease. Approximately 19% of patients who undergo PET are up-staged, whereas only 8% are down-staged. However, because of physiological FDG uptake, cerebral metastases cannot be assessed with sufficient certainty using PET-CT. Therefore, to exclude brain metastases, a cranial CT or MRI scan should be performed in all patients with SCLC within the context of initial staging.

Lung function tests are important to identify patients with poor pulmonary reserve as radical thoracic radiotherapy would be inappropriate for them.

Case history continued

PET-CT confirmed the findings of the CT scan. It showed a pathologically hypermetabolic left upper lobe mass and FDG-avid left paratracheal, precarinal, and subcarinal nodes. No other pathological lesions were observed. Brain MRI demonstrated no central nervous system (CNS) infiltration.

2. What stage is the patient's disease?

Historically, SCLC has been staged using the Veterans Administration Lung Study Group (VALG) classification scheme that defines two stages: limited stage, in which the disease is confined to one hemithorax and can be safely encompassed within a radiation field (both ipsilateral and contralateral hilar, supraclavicular, and mediastinal nodes are generally classified as limited stage), and extensive stage, in which the disease extends beyond the ipsilateral hemithorax, including malignant pleural or pericardial effusion or haematogenous metastases. The seventh edition of the TNM lung cancer classification revised by the International Association for the Study of Lung Cancer (IASLC) and adopted by the Union for International Cancer Control (UICC) recommended the use of this staging system for both non-small-cell lung cancer (NSCLC) and SCLC. This recommendation is based on the studies from the IASLC staging database, which showed that TNM staging provides better prognostic information and more precise nodal staging, which are required for conformal radiation techniques and intensity-modulated radiation therapy. However, the VALG classification is clinically popular because of its usefulness for routine decision-making. Hence, in clinical practice we can generally consider patients with stage I to stage IIIB as having limited stage and stage IV as having extensive stage. The median survival for patients with limited stage disease is currently 15–20 months, with 20–40% surviving to 2 years; for those with extensive stage disease the values are 8–13 months and 5%, respectively.

The patient was staged as T2bN2M0 (stage IIIA).

3. What treatment would you offer to this patient? If you would offer radiation therapy, would you administer it concurrently or sequentially?

Patients with limited stage SCLC and good performance status should be treated with chemotherapy and concurrent thoracic radiotherapy. Although in patients with stage T1–2N0–1M0 surgical resection may be an option, adjuvant chemotherapy is required because of the high risk of relapse following surgery alone.

The most commonly used chemotherapy schedule in fit patients is four to six cycles of combination cisplatin (80 mg/m^2, day 1) and etoposide (100–120 mg/m^2, days 1–3). Carboplatin (area under the curve (AUC) 5) can be used to replace cisplatin in patients for whom cisplatin is contraindicated (poor performance status, renal impairment, peripheral neuropathy, or hearing deficit). This combination is preferred to other regimens containing alkylator or anthracycline based on its greater efficacy and lower toxicity in the limited stage setting.

For extensive disease, the combination of cisplatin and etoposide is also the standard treatment based on the results of two meta-analyses that demonstrated prolonged survival of patients receiving cisplatin and etoposide.

No consistent survival benefit has been shown with increasing dose intensity or dose density with the addition of a third drug to the combination or with maintenance chemotherapy.

Thoracic radiotherapy for limited stage disease yields a 25–30% reduction in local failure and a 7% improvement in 2 year survival compared with chemotherapy alone. Early (beginning with the first or second cycle of chemotherapy) thoracic radiotherapy concurrent with chemotherapy is recommended. The most common radiotherapy schedule is 2.0 Gy once daily to a total dose of 60–70 Gy. The 1.5 Gy twice daily schedule to a total dose of 45 Gy is also used, but with the inconvenience of the administration itself and an increased rate of toxicity. Recently, the CONVERT study comparing once daily (66 Gy in 33 fractions) versus twice daily (45 Gy in 30 fractions) dosing has been reported: the median overall survival and 5 year survival did not differ between the two schedules. Toxicities were comparable and less than expected; only grade 3–4 neutropenia was significantly higher in the twice daily arm.

4. What toxicities would you expect from the treatment?

Oesophagitis as well as pulmonary and haematological toxicities are the most frequent types of toxicity observed with concomitant treatment with cisplatin and etoposide and radiotherapy. The use of myeloid growth factors is usually not recommended in patients receiving concurrent chemoradiotherapy, but can be considered to maintain dose intensity. Carboplatin is used as an alternative to cisplatin in patients not suitable for this and to reduce the risk of emesis, nephropathy, and neuropathy. No difference in outcomes, including response rate, progression-free survival, and overall survival, has been observed between carboplatin and cisplatin. However, the use of carboplatin is associated a higher risk of myelosuppression, whereas an increased risk of renal and neurological toxicity has been found with cisplatin.

Case history continued

The patient was treated with four cycles of cisplatin (80 mg/m², day 1) and etoposide (100 mg/m², days 1–3) every 21 days, plus concomitant once daily radiotherapy (66 Gy in 33 fractions beginning at the second cycle). A CT scan after the treatment showed a partial response: a residual mass of 6 × 5 cm persisted in the left upper lobe with associated atelectasis.

5. Would you recommend any further treatment at this point?

Intracranial metastases occur in more than 50% of patients with SCLC. Prophylactic cranial irradiation (PCI) decreases the incidence of brain metastases and increases survival compared with no PCI. Hence, patients who respond to first-line therapy (limited or extensive stage) and who have a good performance status should be evaluated for PCI.

Case history continued

The patient received PCI (30 Gy in 10 daily fractions) and initiated follow-up. Four months after the end of chemotherapy, the patient complained about right upper abdominal pain. Physical examination noted a large liver with right upper quadrant tenderness. Blood chemistry at the time revealed significantly elevated liver function enzymes, including aspartate aminotransferase (AST) and alanine aminotransferase (ALT). A chest and abdomen CT scan showed stable disease in the chest but the appearance of new hepatic lesions in both liver lobes compatible with metastases.

6. What would you recommend in this situation?

Despite the good response obtained with first-line chemotherapy, most patients relapse or progress with relatively chemoresistant disease. The median survival after progression is only about 4–5 months when treated with further chemotherapy.

Depending on the time from initial therapy to relapse, patients are classified as having refractory or resistant disease, when the interval is <3 months (<10% of patients respond to subsequent therapies), or sensitive disease, when the treatment-free interval is >3 months (the probability of response is about 20%). The sensitive disease group may be divided into sensitive relapse (>3 and <6 months) and late relapse (>6 months) with a more favourable prognosis.

In patients who relapse with a treatment-free interval of <6 months, retreatment with the original platinum–etoposide regimen is recommended. For all patients with refractory, resistant, or sensitive relapse a new drug not used for the first-line therapy should be considered. Topotecan is the therapy of choice in second-line treatment of these patients on the basis of better symptom control and improved survival compared with best supportive care, and is the only licensed drug in this indication. In terms of effectiveness and toxicity, there is no difference between intravenous (1.5 mg/m²) and oral (2.3 mg/m²) administration on days 1–5 in a 21 day cycle.

Prior to topotecan development, anthracycline-based regimes were commonly used, including cyclophosphamide, doxorubicin, and vincristine (CAV), but currently topotecan is preferred because of a similar efficacy to and better tolerance than CAV. However, CAV may remain an alternative to topotecan.

Other active agents in SCLC are irinotecan, amrubicin, docetaxel, paclitaxel, vinorelbine, gemcitabine, and temozolamide, but efficacy data are more limited and third-line chemotherapy for SCLC is rarely used. New agents such as alisertib, an oral selective inhibitor of aurora kinase; immune checkpoint inhibitors (e.g. ipilimumab and nivolumab); and rovalpituzumab tesirine, a targeted agent against Delta-like protein 3 (DLL3), are being investigated in clinical trials, some showing promising activity.

Follow-up and outcome

The patient received six courses of oral topotecan with stable disease at the first and second assessment after the second and third cycles, respectively. After six cycles progressive disease in the liver was observed as well brain metastases. The patient was transferred to the palliative team and died 6 weeks later with good symptom control.

Further reading

Byers LA, Rudin CM. Small cell lung cancer: where do we go from here? Cancer. 2015 Mar;**121**(5):664–72.

Fruh M, De Ruysscher D, Popat S, Crino L, Peters S, Felip E; ESMO Guidelines Working Group. Small-cell lung cancer (SCLC): ESMO Clinical Practice Guidelines for diagnosis, treatment and follow-up. Ann Oncol. 2013 Oct;**24**(Suppl 6):vi99–105.

Kahnert K, Kauffmann-Guerrero D, Huber RM. SCLC—state of the art and what does the future have in store? Clin Lung Cancer. 2016 Sep;**17**(5):325–33.

Koinis F, Kotsakis A, Georgoulias V. Small cell lung cancer (SCLC): no treatment advances in recent years. Transl Lung Cancer Res. 2016 Feb;**5**(1):39–50.

Case 16

Adenocarcinoma identified to be EGFR mutation positive

Oscar Juan and Sanjay Popat

Case history

A 51 year old female presented with a 6 week history of pleuritic chest pain, non-productive cough, and dyspnoea on exertion. She had a 2 month history of asthenia, anorexia, and a 4 kg weight loss. She had never smoked, occasionally consumed alcohol, and had no family history of cancer. Her ECOG performance status was 1. On examination she was dyspnoeic with reduced air entry at the left lung base on auscultation.

A chest x-ray revealed a moderate-sized left pleural effusion. The patient was referred to the chest team, which ordered a chest CT scan that revealed bilateral subcentimetre lung nodules, a large left pleural effusion, pleural deposits, enlarged mediastinal nodes, bone metastases, and multiple small liver metastases (<1 cm). The patient underwent thoracocentesis with removal of nearly 1.5 L of straw-coloured fluid. The pleural fluid was positive for malignant cells, suggestive of adenocarcinoma.

Questions

1. Which immunohistochemistry profile would be consistent with a diagnosis of adenocarcinoma of the lung?
2. Which molecular tests would you recommend based upon available guidelines for this patient?
3. What is the most appropriate next step?
4. Which first-line treatment would you recommend for this patient?
5. What are considered to be the common EGFR mutations? Is the same response observed across different types of EGFR mutations?
6. Are adverse events different according to the type of EGFR TKI?
7. What would you do at this point?
8. Which is the most appropriate treatment option for this patient at this time?
9. Would liquid biopsy be adequate for this patient instead of rebiopsy?
10. What is the most appropriate next step when a T790M mutation is negative using a ctDNA EGFR test?
11. What is the safety profile of osimertinib?
12. Which mechanisms of resistance have been observed following treatment with osimertinib?

Answers

1. Which immunohistochemistry profile would be consistent with a diagnosis of adenocarcinoma of the lung?

Positive cytokeratin-7 (CK7) and thyroid transcription factor-1 (TTF-1) is the profile most consistent with adenocarcinoma. TTF-1 is positive in nearly 75% of lung adenocarcinomas and it seems to confer a favourable prognosis in survival compared with TTF-1-negative adenocarcinoma patients. Primary lung tumours are also positive for CK7 and negative for CK20. Positivity for CK20 is suggestive of intestinal tract origin. Otherwise, p63 is positive in the majority of squamous cell carcinomas (SCCs) of the lung.

Case history continued

With the above immunohistochemistry (IHC) findings a diagnosis of adenocarcinoma of the lung stage T4N2M1b (stage IV) was made.

2. Which molecular tests would you recommend based upon available guidelines for this patient?

Assessment of epidermal growth factor receptor (EGFR) mutation and anaplastic lymphoma kinase (ALK) gene rearrangement for all patients with advanced stage adenocarcinoma of the lung is recommended for this patient according to most clinical guidelines (IASLC, European Society of Medical Oncology (ESMO), American Society of Clinical Oncology (ASCO)). Although routine testing for other biomarkers is not currently recommended, next-generation sequencing could be considered and is increasingly popular since other biomarkers, for which potential active agents are already approved for other indications, have been identified. These biomarkers include ROS proto-oncogene 1 receptor tyrosine kinase (ROS-1) and RET proto-oncogene gene rearrangements, erb-b2 receptor tyrosine kinase 2 (HER2) amplifications and mutation, B-Raf proto-oncogene serine/threonine kinase (BRAF) mutations, and MET proto-oncogene receptor tyrosine kinase mutations.

Case history continued

The patient's cytology specimen did not contain adequate cells to conduct molecular analysis.

3. What is the most appropriate next step?

Chemotherapy could be recommended if the patient was unstable or if a biopsy was considered unsafe because of the location of the tumour. In all other cases, when the specimen for molecular testing is inadequate, a repeat biopsy is indicated to determine EGFR and ALK status.

Case history continued

Thoracoscopy with pleural biopsy and talc pleurodesis was performed. Biopsies confirmed a TTF-1-positive adenocarcinoma. Molecular analysis of a biopsy specimen identified an exon 19 deletion in the EGFR gene. ALK rearrangement was negative.

4. Which first-line treatment would you recommend for this patient?

The EGFR tyrosine kinase inhibitors (TKIs) afatinib, erlotinib, or gefitinib are considered standard first-line therapy for patients with EGFR-activating mutations. In phase III studies all of these agents have demonstrated an improvement in response rate and progression-free survival compared with chemotherapy in EGFR mutation-positive patients. In patients with typical EGFR common mutations treated with EGFR TKIs the median response rate was 50–70% and the median progression-free survival was 9–13 months.

Although no significant difference in overall survival was observed between treatment arms, the median survival was >22 months in patients treated with EGFR TKIs. One of the possible reasons for not observing a survival gain after a progression-free survival improvement is the influence of postprogression therapy. In the phase III trials comparing EGFR TKIs with chemotherapy, crossover is a huge confounder for overall survival due to 57–98% of patients assigned to the chemotherapy arm receiving second- or third-line therapy with EGFR TKIs.

5. What are considered to be the common EGFR mutations? Is the same response observed across different types of EGFR mutations?

Activating EGFR somatic mutations are mainly observed in exons 18–21, which encode part of the tyrosine kinase domain of the gene and are clustered around the ATP-binding pocket. The most common EGFR mutations are exon 19 deletions (del19) and exon 21 L858R substitutions (45–82% and 30%, respectively), which are commonly referred to as *sensitizing mutations* as they confer sensitivity to TKIs and constitute approximately 80–90% of EGFR mutations in adenocarcinomas. Sensitizing mutations in exon 18 (G719C, G719S, G719A, and S720F) and others in exon 21 (L861Q and L861R) are less common. Other mutations include exon 20 insertions and point mutations, which are associated with primary TKI resistance.

Whether the efficacy of EGFR TKIs varies between the two common mutations (del19 and L858R) is controversial. Several studies and meta-analyses have shown a greater benefit in terms of progression-free survival in patients with EGFR del19 than in those with L858R. The greatest difference between these two groups of patients has been observed with afatinib.

Data regarding the sensitivity of tumours harbouring uncommon EGFR mutations such as E709X, G719X, L861Q, S768I, and others to TKIs are limited because most phase III trials compare first-line TKIs with chemotherapy and are restricted to common mutations (del19/L858R). The largest dataset for uncommon mutations comes from studies with afatinib. For the most frequent uncommon mutations, the objective response rate (ORR) was 77.8% for G719X, 56.3% for L861Q, and 100% for S768I.

6. Are adverse events different according to the type of EGFR TKI?

Trial results suggest that the toxicity profiles of TKIs are different. Grade 3–4 diarrhoea and stomatitis are more frequent for afatinib; rash or acne more frequent for erlotinib; whereas increased ALT/AST levels are more common for gefitinib. The frequency of grade ≥3 interstitial lung disease was low and similar between all three EGFR TKIs.

Case history continued

The patient started treatment with gefitinib at a dose of 250 mg daily. She tolerated the drug very well. A CT scan demonstrated a very good partial response with an 85% reduction in lung lesions and disappearance of liver metastases.

The patient was continued on therapy with gefitinib for 19 months until she complained about right upper abdominal pain. A CT scan revealed stable disease in the lung but larger hepatic lesions (Fig. 16.1).

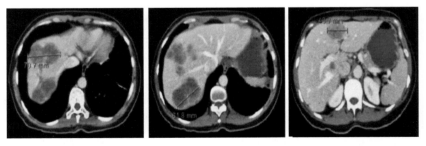

Fig. 16.1 CT scan of the liver showing progression of the metastatic disease (right to left).

7. What would you do at this point?

Despite the good response and prolonged progression-free survival observed with EGFR TKI therapy, virtually all patients progress because of acquired resistance. The most frequent molecular mechanism of acquired resistance observed is the development of the gatekeeper T790M point mutation in EGFR (observed in up to 60% of cases). However, other mechanisms such as MET amplification, HER2 amplification, and even small-cell transformation have been described (Fig. 16.2).

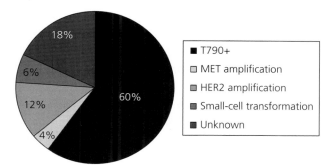

Fig. 16.2 Mechanisms of acquired resistance to EGFR TKIs.

Asymptomatic patients with slow progression and low tumour burden may continue with the same EGFR TKI. However, in this patient with large liver metastases and rapid disease progression a biopsy is recommended to identify the cause of her resistance.

Case history continued

Rebiopsy of the liver metastases was performed. Molecular testing revealed the presence of the EGFR del19 and T790M mutations.

8. Which is the most appropriate treatment option for this patient at this time?

For patients with documented T790M mutations, the US Food and Drug Administration (FDA) and the European Medicines Agency (EMA) have recently approved the third-generation TKI osimertinib. In T790M-positive patients, osimertinib has shown a 61% ORR and 9.6 month progression-free survival. In contrast, in T790M-negative patients, ORR was 21% and progression-free survival was

2.8 months. For this reason osimertinib is not recommended in the absence of the T790M mutation. Chemotherapy can be considered in patients with disease progression shown to be T790M negative from a representative new biopsy.

9. Would liquid biopsy be adequate for this patient instead of rebiopsy?

Circulating tumour DNA (ctDNA) can be an alternative for T790M testing. It has high specificity but low sensitivity compared with tissue EGFR status. In approximately 30% of patients with a T790M mutation, the plasma test can be negative. Studies have shown that the ORR to treatment with osimertinib in patients who were tumour and plasma T790M positive was 62% and 63%, respectively. However, the ORR in T790M-negative tumours was 26%, whereas in patients with T790M-negative plasma the ORR was 46%, implying false negative results from the plasma test.

10. What is the most appropriate next step when a T790M mutation is negative using a ctDNA EGFR test?

Since plasma test sensitivity is approximately 70%, a tumour biopsy is indicated. Moreover, in the case of T790M mutation-negative patients, other mechanisms of acquired resistance with implications for the treatment of patients such as the small-cell carcinoma transformation may be identified. However, for most patients with T790M-negative disease, other than clinical trials, platinum doublet chemotherapy is the most appropriate choice in this setting.

Case history continued

The patient started treatment with osimertinib 80 mg daily with excellent tolerance. A CT scan performed at 6 weeks revealed the disappearance of the lung nodules and an important reduction in liver metastases (Fig. 16.3).

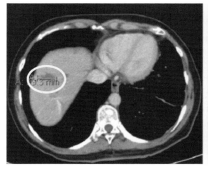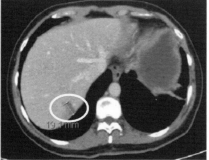

Fig. 16.3 CT scan of the liver showing a reduction in the size of the liver metastasis compared with the CT scan of the liver in Fig. 16.1.

11. What is the safety profile of osimertinib?

The commonest grade 3 and grade 4 adverse events are skin rash and diarrhoea in less than 5% of patients treated with 80 mg osimertinib daily. Rare cases of pneumonitis have been observed.

Other third-generation TKIs such as rociletinib and olmutinib have been tested in this scenario; however, they are no longer being developed because of efficacy and toxicity results in initial trials.

Case history continued

The patient was treated with osimertinib for 30 months and maintained a good response with ECOG performance status 0. A CT scan revealed new liver and bone lesions.

12. Which mechanisms of resistance have been observed following treatment with osimertinib?

In nearly one-third of patients treated with osimertinib a new EGFR C797S mutation has been demonstrated as a resistance mechanism. This mutation occurs at the binding site where osimertinib forms a covalent bond with the EGFR. Bypass tract signalling such as KRAS G12S and transformation to SCLC have also been described as other resistance mechanisms.

Further reading

Chouaid C et al. Feasibility and clinical impact of re-biopsy in advanced non-small-cell lung cancer: a prospective multicenter study in a real-world setting (GFPC study 12-01). Lung Cancer. 2014 Nov;**86**(2):170–3.

Felip E et al. Biomarker testing in advanced non-small-cell lung cancer: a National Consensus of the Spanish Society of Pathology and the Spanish Society of Medical Oncology. Clin Transl Oncol. 2015 Feb;**17**(2):103–12.

Novello S et al. Metastatic non-small-cell lung cancer: ESMO Clinical Practice Guidelines for diagnosis, treatment and follow-up. Ann Oncol. 2016 Sep;**27**(Suppl 5):v1–v27.

Oxnard GR, Thress KS, Alden RS, Lawrance R, Paweletz CP, Cantarini M, Yang JC, Barrett JC, Jänne PA. Association between plasma genotyping and outcomes of treatment with osimertinib (AZD9291) in advanced non-small-cell lung cancer. J Clin Oncol. 2016 Oct;**34**(28):3375–82.

Yu HA et al. Analysis of tumor specimens at the time of acquired resistance to EGFR-TKI therapy in 155 patients with EGFR-mutant lung cancers. Clin Cancer Res. 2013 Apr;**19**(8):2240–7.

Case 17

Adenocarcinoma identified to be ALK fusion positive

Oscar Juan and Sanjay Popat

Case history

A 40 year old female with no history of smoking presented with three thrombotic events over the previous 6 months. Physical examination was non-contributory. She had no previous relevant history and her ECOG performance status was 0. Chest x-ray showed a mass in the lower lobe of the left lung. Bronchoscopy was unremarkable.

PET-CT scan showed a hypermetabolic mass >5 cm in the left lung with a maximum standard uptake value (SUV_{max}) of 10.2 g/mL, accompanied by multiple mediastinal adenopathy measuring ≤1 cm with an SUV_{max} of 8 g/mL (Fig. 17.1). Hypermetabolic bone lytic lesions were observed (Fig. 17.2).

The patient underwent a biopsy of the lung mass, which confirmed a TTF-1-positive adenocarcinoma. A brain MRI was negative for malignancy. Based on these findings a diagnosis of adenocarcinoma of the lung T2bN3M1b (stage IVB) was made.

Questions

1. What molecular testing would you recommend for this patient?
2. What is the gold standard method of detecting an ALK rearrangement?
3. What treatment would you recommend for this patient at this point?
4. How would you manage this patient?
5. What treatment would you recommend for this patient at this point?

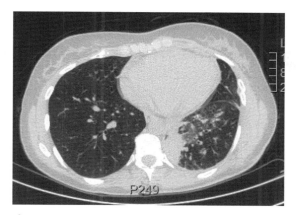

Fig. 17.1 A 5 cm mass located in the left lower lobe.

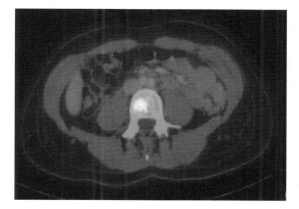

Fig. 17.2 The vertebral body of L4 with an SUV$_{max}$ of 7.1 g/mL, suggesting spinal metastasis.

Answers

1. What molecular testing would you recommend for this patient?

ESMO guidelines recommend the assessment of EGFR mutations and ALK gene rearrangements for all patients with advanced stage adenocarcinoma of the lung.

Other biomarkers such as ROS-1 and RET rearrangements, MET or HER2 amplifications or mutations, and BRAF or phosphatidylinositol-4,5-bisphosphate 3-kinase catalytic subunit alpha (PIK3CA) mutations are not recommended as routine testing, but potential active agents for these biomarkers have been approved for other indications. Next-generation sequencing is becoming more available and allows the assessment of multiple genes on the same sample at the same time.

Case history continued

Molecular testing revealed that the tumour was EGFR wild type (mutation negative) and confirmed the presence of an ALK rearrangement (ALK positive).

2. What is the gold standard method of detecting an ALK rearrangement?

Rearrangement of the ALK gene occurs in approximately 5% of lung adenocarcinomas. The Vysis ALK Break Apart FISH Probe Kit is the gold standard diagnostic test for detecting ALK. However, fluorescence in situ hybridization (FISH) can be expensive and time-consuming and requires specialized fluorescence microscopy equipment and expertise because of difficulties in interpreting the results. As a result, high interobserver variability as well as false negative and false positive results have been observed.

New ALK monoclonal antibody clones (e.g. 5A4) can accurately predict for ALK rearrangement in lung adenocarcinomas by IHC, with 93% sensitivity and 100% specificity.

As false negative and false positive cases exist with both techniques, the recommendation is to examine the ALK gene by both methods when uncertainties of any kind exist regarding the test result.

3. What treatment would you recommend for this patient at this point?

Patients with advanced NSCLC harbouring the ALK rearrangement are highly sensitive to treatment with ALK TKIs such as crizotinib. In a phase III trial in ALK-positive patients with metastatic NSCLC previously treated with chemotherapy, crizotinib compared with second-line chemotherapy showed a significantly increased progression-free survival (median 7.7 versus 3 months) and response rate (60% versus 20%). No significant difference in overall survival was observed (median 20.3 versus 22.8 months), mainly because 64% of chemotherapy-treated patients received crizotinib after progressing.

In a second trial conducted in chemotherapy-naive ALK-positive patients, progression-free survival was also significantly prolonged with crizotinib compared with chemotherapy (median 10.9 versus 7 months). On the basis of the results of these trials crizotinib is preferred as the initial therapy for patients with tumours containing an ALK rearrangement. Thus, ALK testing should be performed at the point of diagnosis. Since ALK rearrangements are almost universally restricted to adenocarcinomas, current guidelines recommend the testing of non-squamous NSCLC.

Case history continued

The patient started treatment with crizotinib 250 mg twice daily. Tolerability was good and a CT scan performed at 2 months showed an excellent partial response (Fig. 17.3). The patient continued crizotinib but 10 months later complained about thoracic pain. A CT scan showed progression of the lung mass with no other lesions. Bone scan did not reveal any progressive disease.

4. How would you manage this patient?

The traditional approach when there is objective evidence of clinical or radiological progression is to discontinue or change systemic therapy. However, in patients with EGFR mutations or ALK rearrangements who progress in only a limited number of sites (oligoprogressive disease) after a previous benefit, one can consider local therapy to sites of progression with continuation of the TKI. This strategy is associated with more than 6 months of additional disease control. An alternative is to switch systemic therapy.

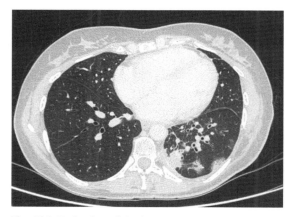

Fig. 17.3 Reduction of the lung mass.

Case history continued

The patient was treated with stereotactic body radiation therapy and continued with crizotinib. Twelve months later she presented with new progression in the treated lung lesion (Fig. 17.4) and in the bone metastases.

5. What treatment would you recommend for this patient at this point?

Almost all patients treated with crizotinib develop resistance to the drug through inadequate ALK inhibition, acquisition of a secondary mutation, amplification of the ALK fusion gene, or a number of alternative or bypass signalling pathways. Several second- or third-generation highly potent ALK inhibitors such as ceritinib, alectinib, brigatinib, and lorlatinib have activity in crizotinib-resistant disease.

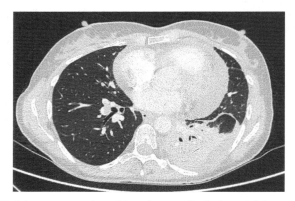

Fig. 17.4 Lung progression with an increase in the lung left lower mass.

Follow-up and outcome

The patient was treated with ceritinib, with a further excellent partial response, and remains on therapy (5 months).

Further reading

Ou SHI et al. Clinical benefit of continuing ALK inhibition with crizotinib beyond initial disease progression in patients with advanced ALK-positive NSCLC. Ann Oncol. 2014 Feb;**25**(2):415–22.

Shaw AT, **Solomon B**. Targeting anaplastic lymphoma kinase in lung cancer. Clin Cancer Res. 2011 Apr;**17**(8):2081–6.

Shaw AT et al. Crizotinib versus chemotherapy in advanced ALK-positive lung cancer. N Engl J Med. 2013 Jun;**368**(25):2385–94.

Solomon BJ et al. First-line crizotinib versus chemotherapy in ALK-positive lung cancer. N Engl J Med. 2014 Dec;**371**(23):2167–77.

Weickhardt AJ et al. Local ablative therapy of oligoprogressive disease prolongs disease control by tyrosine kinase inhibitors in oncogene-addicted non-small-cell lung cancer. J Thorac Oncol. 2012 Dec;**7**(12):1807–14.

Case 18

Relapsed stage IV adenocarcinoma with insufficient material for genotyping at diagnosis

Nadza Tokaca and Sanjay Popat

Case history

A 50 year old female underwent lobectomy for pT2bN0M0, TTF-1-positive adeno-carcinoma of the lung in 2013. She was treated thereafter with adjuvant chemo-therapy of four cycles of cisplatin and vinorelbine; she then underwent routine surveillance. A CT scan of the thorax and abdomen performed 9 months after completion of adjuvant chemotherapy identified multiple (>3) small bilateral new lung nodules in the right upper and left lower lobes of the lung and mediastinal lymphadenopathy (Fig. 18.1a,b). Endobronchial ultrasound (EBUS) was performed and confirmed a relapsed metastatic TTF-1-positive adenocarcinoma. Molecular analysis of EGFR and ALK failed because of insufficient tumour material in the diag-nostic specimen. The patient was currently mildly symptomatic with dyspnoea on moderate exertion and an ECOG performance status of 1.

Questions

1. What other information about the patient's history is needed?
2. What would be the most appropriate next step in this patient's management?
3. What investigations would you consider at this time?
4. What investigations would you request at this point?
5. What systemic management options would you consider?

(a)

(b)

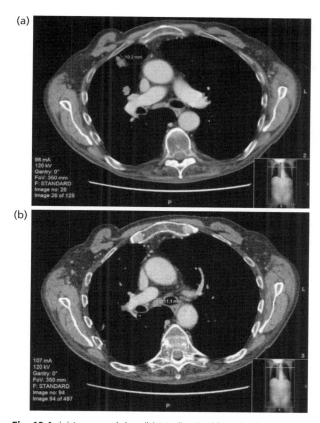

Fig. 18.1 (a) Lung nodules. (b) Mediastinal lymphadenopathy.

Answers

1. What other information about the patient's history is needed?

The patient's smoking history is needed.

Case history continued

The patient had a history of light ex-smoking (5 pack-years), having stopped at the age of 30.

---

2. What would be the most appropriate next step in this patient's management?

Rebiopsy should be considered. If tissue rebiopsy is not feasible, EGFR genotyping by plasma ctDNA testing should be considered.

Case history continued

The case was rediscussed at the multidisciplinary team (MDT) meeting and no other feasible rebiopsy sites were identified. ctDNA EGFR genotyping was requested and did not identify an EGFR mutation. The patient was commenced on palliative systemic chemotherapy with cisplatin and pemetrexed; however, a response assessment CT scan after two cycles of treatment showed disease progression due to growth in many of the lung metastases and a new contrast-enhancing liver lesion consistent with a metastasis.

---

3. What investigations would you consider at this time?

An ultrasound (US)-guided biopsy of the liver should be carried out to obtain tissue for molecular analysis of the EGFR and ALK genes. Broader molecular analysis for other emerging biomarkers, including ROS-1 and RET rearrangements and BRAF, should also be considered.

Case history continued

A US-guided liver biopsy yielded sufficient tissue to confirm a TTF-1-positive adenocarcinoma. EGFR and ALK testing confirmed the presence of an EGFR-activating mutation in exon 19 (deletion). The patient was commenced on afatinib 40 mg once daily with an excellent partial response on CT after two cycles of treatment. After 9 months on afatinib, a CT chest/abdomen scan showed progressive disease with multiple new liver metastases.

4. What investigations would you request at this point?

Tissue rebiopsy, if feasible, should be requested. ctDNA testing for the EGFR T790M mutation should also be considered.

Role of rebiopsy, including molecular yield, and non-invasive methods, i.e. ctDNA

Routine molecular tumour characterization at diagnosis is recommended for all patients with relapsed or metastatic non-squamous NSCLC in order to guide the optimal choice of first-line treatment for metastatic disease. Predictive molecular biomarkers in NSCLC include sensitizing EGFR mutations (typically exon 19 deletions and the exon 21 L858R point mutation) and ALK fusions. Sensitizing EGFR mutations occur in around 10% of Western patients with NSCLC and are predictive of treatment benefit with the EGFR TKIs gefitinib, erlotinib, and afatinib. ALK rearrangements occur in around 5% of patients and are predictive of responses to the ALK TKI crizotinib. A number of other emerging biomarkers have been identified that indicate susceptibility to targeted therapies, including HER2 and BRAF V600E mutations, ROS-1 and RET gene rearrangements, high-level MET amplification, or MET exon 14 skipping mutations. Thus, broader molecular profiling is desirable to identify rare driver mutations and to ensure that patients receive the most appropriate treatments and/or confirm eligibility for clinical trials of targeted agents. Next-generation sequencing can be used for testing of an entire panel of gene mutations at a single time from a single tissue sample, although, contingent on the technology used, this may not be suitable for detecting gene rearrangements.

When the initial diagnostic tissue is inadequate for molecular testing, a rebiopsy should be considered to obtain additional material prior to commencing systemic treatment. The most commonly used sampling techniques include percutaneous core needle biopsy, EBUS with transbronchial needle aspiration, and conventional bronchoscopy with forceps biopsy. The choice of tissue sampling technique is critical for subsequent molecular profiling and primarily depends on the tumour location and local expertise. Fine needle aspiration is minimally invasive and may have safety advantages, although a core needle biopsy provides larger tissue samples that may be considered more reliable and informative. Both techniques are capable of generating adequate material for molecular and diagnostic tests.

If rebiopsy is not feasible, a validated alternative to tissue biopsy is a 'liquid biopsy', in which plasma samples are collected for ctDNA extraction and genotyping. Compared with tissue EGFR genotyping, ctDNA EGFR genotyping has been shown to be highly specific but not hugely sensitive. It is clinically recommended in patients with a proven EGFR mutation with acquired resistance to afatinib, erlotinib, or gefitinib.

In the event of an EGFR T790M mutation being detected on ctDNA testing (or tissue biopsy), treatment with the third-generation mutation-specific EGFR TKI osimertinib may be indicated. If the T790M mutation is not identified on ctDNA analysis, because of the low sensitivity, a tissue rebiopsy is recommended if feasible.

5. What systemic management options would you consider?

In the presence of disease progression and identification of the EGFR T790M acquired resistance mutation (either on tissue rebiopsy or ctDNA analysis), consideration of switching treatment to the mutation-specific EGFR TKI osimertinib should be given. If the T790M mutation is not detected on ctDNA analysis or tissue biopsy, consideration should be given to switching to systemic chemotherapy (e.g. docetaxel with or without nintedanib).

Treatment options for molecularly defined subsets

Patients whose tumours harbour a driver mutation should receive appropriate targeted treatments as initial therapy for advanced disease. For patients with activating EGFR mutations, the EGFR TKIs gefitinib, erlotinib, and afatinib represent the standard of care for first-line therapy. Afatinib achieves higher response rates and progression-free survival than gefitinib and is the only EGFR TKI to demonstrate improved overall survival compared with first-line chemotherapy, albeit only in patients with the EGFR exon 19 deletion mutation and not in those with the L858R mutation.

If EGFR sensitizing mutation information becomes available during first-line treatment with platinum doublet chemotherapy, patients should receive second-line EGFR TKI treatment on progression.

Most patients will progress after a median of 9–12 months on first-line TKI therapy. Such patients should undergo a tissue rebiopsy, or liquid rebiopsy if a tissue rebiopsy is not feasible, to look for the presence of the EGFR T790M mutation. This is the commonest mechanism of acquired EGFR TKI resistance and can be found in around 50% of patients at the time of disease progression. Patients confirmed to have an EGFR T790M mutation should receive osimertinib, an oral, selective, third-generation, irreversible EGFR TKI with activity against the T790M mutation. When the EGFR T790M mutation is not detected as a resistance mechanism, the standard of care is platinum-based chemotherapy alone. There is no evidence to support continuation of the EGFR TKI with platinum-based chemotherapy.

There is evidence that in those patients with radiological progression at a single site (i.e. CNS metastasis or adrenal gland), but with ongoing dependence on the driver oncogene addiction and without rapid systemic progression, local ablative treatment (radiotherapy or surgery) with continuation of the EGFR TKI may represent a reasonable option and should be considered.

The first-line treatment in ALK-rearranged patients is crizotinib, a dual ALK and MET TKI. First-line therapy with crizotinib improves progression-free survival, response rate, lung cancer symptoms, and quality of life when compared with chemotherapy (pemetrexed with either cisplatin or carboplatin). Upon progression on crizotinib, second-line treatment with the second-generation ALK TKI ceritinib is recommended. Newer ALK inhibitors, characterized by broader activity against a range of ALK aberrations and higher brain activity, are in development (alectinib, brigatinib).

Evidence for targeted therapies in patients with other genetic alterations is emerging (Table 18.1). Crizotinib has recently been licensed in patients with ROS-1 rearrangements and has shown efficacy in MET amplifications or MET exon 14 mutations. Other new targets include BRAF V600E mutations and RET rearrangements. Patients with these molecular aberrations should be considered for clinical trial enrolment when licensed therapies are not available.

Table 18.1 Emerging targets in NSCLC

Driver event in NSCLC	Targeted agents with activity against driver event
BRAF V600E mutation	Vemurafenib Dabrafenib Dabrafenib + trametinib
High-level MET amplification or MET exon 14 skipping mutation	Crizotinib
RET rearrangements	Cabozantinib Vandetanib
ROS-1 rearrangements	Crizotinib

Treatment options for biomarker-negative non-squamous NSCLC

The standard-of-care initial therapy for patients with metastatic NSCLC without a driver mutation is platinum-based doublet chemotherapy for four to six cycles. Pemetrexed in combination with platinum has shown survival benefit over gemcitabine- or docetaxel-based combinations and is the preferred option in non-squamous NSCLC.

For patients aged >70 years or with reduced ECOG performance status (performance status ≥2), carboplatin instead of cisplatin doublet- or single-agent chemotherapy (gemcitabine, vinorelbine, or docetaxel) should be considered.

The addition of bevacizumab to platinum-based doublet chemotherapy may improve survival in patients with non-squamous NSCLC and ECOG performance status 0–1 and is an option in the absence of contraindications.

Maintenance therapy should be considered in patients with a good performance status who achieve a response or who have stable disease after platinum-based therapy. This could consist of pemetrexed (switch maintenance or continuation maintenance if given before) or erlotinib with or without bevacizumab if given before.

Based on the results from a recent phase III trial of the anti-programmed cell death-1 (PD-1) antibody pembrolizumab versus platinum-based chemotherapy in treatment-naive patients with advanced NSCLC, pembrolizumab has been approved by the FDA for first-line use in patients whose tumours have high expression of programmed cell death ligand-1 (PD-L1) and no driver mutations in their tumours.

On progression after first-line therapy, the treatment options for non-squamous NSCLC in patients with no driver mutations include single-agent chemotherapy with docetaxel with the addition of the angiokinase inhibitor nintedanib; single-agent pemetrexed if not given in the first line; or immunotherapy with nivolumab, pembrolizumab, or atezolizumab. Nivolumab showed improved survival benefit compared with docetaxel in patients positive for the PD-L1 biomarker, and a similar benefit to docetaxel in PD-L1-negative patients, with a lower frequency of serious adverse events. Treatment with pembrolizumab requires tumour expression of the PD-L1 biomarker >1%.

Learning points

◆ All patients with relapsed or metastatic non-squamous NSCLC should have routine testing of EGFR and ALK at diagnosis.

◆ Tissue rebiopsy should be performed when feasible if the initial diagnostic biopsy is inadequate for molecular analysis.

◆ Liquid biopsy is a validated alternative to tissue biopsy if tissue biopsy is not feasible.

◆ In EGFR-mutated patients, repeat rebiopsy and/or liquid biopsy for EGFR T790M testing should be considered on progression on first-line EGFR TKI therapy.

◆ Broader molecular testing for emerging biomarkers is desirable for optimal management.

Further reading

Jiang T, Ren S, Zhou C. Role of circulating-tumor DNA analysis in non-small cell lung cancer. Lung Cancer. 2015 Nov;**90**(2):128–34.

Moreira AL, Thornton RH. Personalized medicine for non-small-cell lung cancer: implications of recent advances in tissue acquisition for molecular and histologic testing. Clin Lung Cancer. 2012 Sep;**13**(5):334–9.

National Comprehensive Cancer Network. Non-Small Cell Lung Cancer. National Comprehensive Cancer Network Guidelines in Oncology, Version 2.2017, published 26 October 2016. Fort Washington, PA: National Comprehensive Cancer Network. Available at https://www.nccn.org/professionals

Novello S et al. Metastatic non-small-cell lung cancer: ESMO Clinical Practice Guidelines for diagnosis, treatment and follow-up. Ann Oncol. 2016 Sep;**27**(Suppl 5):v1–v27.

Case 19

Squamous cell carcinoma of the lung in a patient with previous breast cancer

Spyros Gennatas and Sanjay Popat

Case history

A 67 year old female presented to an accident and emergency department with haemoptysis. She had been well until 2 days prior, when she had had another episode of haemoptysis. She was planning to see her GP but, as the next available appointment was 12 days later, following a second episode of haemoptysis she decided to go to the hospital. Three years earlier she had had a right-sided mastectomy for a stage IIB invasive ductal carcinoma (pT3pN0M0, triple negative—oestrogen receptor, progesterone receptor, and HER2 negative) breast cancer. She had been a smoker since her teens, accumulating a 50 pack-year history. She also had a history of chronic obstructive pulmonary disease (COPD), which was under good control with the use of inhaled steroids and bronchodilators. She did not have any other complaints apart from a mild irritating cough; she also admitted that she had lost her appetite over recent weeks and felt her trousers were a bit looser.

On examination she was slightly tachypnoeic with a respiratory rate of 23/min and her oxygen saturation was 95% on room air. Auscultation of her chest revealed a mild bilateral wheeze. A set of routine blood tests revealed a slightly raised white cell count at 14×10^9/L with neutrophilia. A chest x-ray was performed, which revealed a right-sided mass with probable bilateral pulmonary nodules (Fig. 19.1).

Questions

1. What would be the investigation of choice at this stage?
2. What is the likely diagnosis and how can it be confirmed?
3. What other information do you need to know before starting to treat this patient?
4. How would you treat this patient?

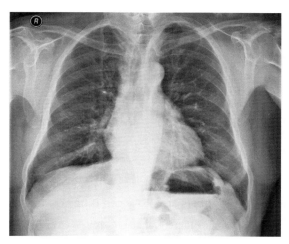

Fig. 19.1 Chest x-ray at presentation showing a right lower lobe mass.

Answers

1. What would be the investigation of choice at this stage?

A CT scan of the chest, abdomen, and pelvis would be the investigation of choice at this stage. In this patient, the CT scan confirmed the presence of multiple pulmonary nodules bilaterally, with one larger dominant spiculated lung mass. There was a rim of pericardial effusion and a suspicious lesion on the left adrenal gland that could not be adequately characterized on CT alone. The findings were reported as consistent with metastatic disease with lung being the most likely primary site.

2. What is the likely diagnosis and how can it be confirmed?

With the above information the differential diagnosis lies between a new metastatic lung malignancy, breast cancer recurrence, and metastatic disease from another primary not visualized on CT. The presence of an adrenal lesion, although indeterminate, increases the probability of this being a lung primary.

A tissue diagnosis is therefore essential to establish the primary site and determine the exact histology of the likely malignancy. Bronchoscopic or percutaneous methods can be used to obtain good quality tissue.

Case history continued

A transbronchial biopsy was performed and revealed a p63- and CK5/6-positive carcinoma with typical squamous features. Given the CT findings, the MDT concluded a diagnosis of stage IV squamous subtype NSCLC by virtue of the bilateral lung nodules, the likely lung primary identified on CT, and the likely pericardial effusion with or without adrenal involvement.

3. What other information do you need to know before starting to treat this patient?

EGFR mutations and ALK rearrangements are currently the only genetic alterations in NSCLC for which there are approved first-line targeted therapies. However, given that these are rare in SCC, mutation testing is only recommended in never or ex-light smokers (<15 pack-years). In the absence of any of these mutations, tumours that have ≥50% of cells expressing PD-L1 can be treated with frontline immune checkpoint inhibitor therapy.

For patients with advanced NSCLC and PD-L1 expression on at least 50% of their tumour cells, the anti-PD-1 antibody pembrolizumab is recommended. This has recently been shown to be associated with significantly longer progression-free survival and overall survival compared with platinum-based doublet chemotherapy. Pembrolizumab also has a better side-effect profile.

The recent development of immune checkpoint inhibitors has revolutionized the treatment of many solid tumours. There are numerous immune checkpoints, which trigger inhibitory pathways that restrict immune responses and help tumours avoid being recognized and attacked by the immune system. The pathway that has currently been exploited the most in NSCLC is the PD-1/PD-L1 pathway. Two agents have been licensed for use in SCC of the lung: nivolumab and pembrolizumab.

Nivolumab is an immunoglobulin (Ig)G4 monoclonal antibody to PD-1 that has received FDA and EMA approval as second-line treatment upon progression following platinum-based chemotherapy for the treatment of squamous and non-squamous NSCLC. In SCC of the lung the phase III CheckMate 017 trial compared second-line nivolumab (3 mg/kg i.v. every 2 weeks) with docetaxel (75 mg/m^2 i.v. every 3 weeks) and showed a prolonged median overall survival with nivolumab (9.2 months (95% confidence interval (CI) 7.3–13.3 months) versus 6.0 months (95% CI 5.1–7.3 months)). These results were seen irrespective of tumour PD-L1 protein expression, which was neither prognostic nor predictive of the clinical benefit seen. Grade 3 or higher toxicities were less frequent with nivolumab.

In the first-line setting the CheckMate 026 trial on advanced PD-L1-positive NSCLC (>1% tumour cells with PD-L1 staining) compared nivolumab (3 mg/kg every 2 weeks) with standard first-line platinum-based doublet chemotherapy but did not show a progression-free survival or overall survival advantage. Nivolumab is therefore not considered for first-line decision-making in SCC of the lung.

Pembrolizumab, another IgG4 anti-PD-1 monoclonal antibody, has also been given FDA and EMA approval for the treatment of any NSCLC at the second-line setting based on the results of the phase II/III KEYNOTE-010 study that assigned patients with >1% tumour cell PD-L1 expression to pembrolizumab 2 mg/kg, pembrolizumab 10 mg/kg, or docetaxel. Median overall survival was improved in all patients (10.4 and 12.7 months versus 8.5 months for the docetaxel-treated group (hazard ratio (HR) 0.71, 95% CI 0.58–0.88 and 0.61, 95% CI 0.49–0.75, respectively)). The results were even more impressive among patients with >50% of tumour cells expressing PD-L1: for those treated with pembrolizumab 2 mg/kg and 10 mg/kg, median overall survival of 14.9 months and 17.3 months, respectively, versus 8.2 months for the docetaxel group (HR 0.54, 95% CI 0.38–0.77 and 0.50, 95% CI 0.36–0.70, respectively). Grade 3 or higher toxicities were less common with pembrolizumab. The current recommended dose is 2 mg/kg administered as an intravenous infusion every 3 weeks.

In the first-line setting in the phase III KEYNOTE-024 study pembrolizumab was compared with standard platinum-based doublet chemotherapy in patients with advanced NSCLC with >50% tumour cells expressing PD-L1 who did not have EGFR mutations or ALK translocations. Here, the pembrolizumab dosing was a 200 mg flat dose every 3 weeks. Progression-free survival was prolonged with pembrolizumab versus chemotherapy (median progression-free survival 10.3

versus 6 months; HR 0.50, 95% CI 0.37–0.68). The estimated rate of overall survival at 6 months was 80.2% in the pembrolizumab group versus 72.4% in the chemotherapy group (HR for death 0.60, 95% CI 0.41–0.89, $P = 0.005$). Severe grade 3–5 toxicities were seen less frequently in the immunotherapy group.

Case history continued

In this case the patient's tumour had only 25% tumour cell PD-L1 staining.

4. How would you treat this patient?

Platinum-based doublet chemotherapy with palliative intent is recommended for stage IV SCC of the lung.

First-line chemotherapy for advanced SCC of the lung

Platinum-based doublet chemotherapy should be considered in all patients with stage IV NSCLC with EGFR- and ALK-negative disease and an ECOG performance status of 0–2. Two meta-analyses have shown the benefit of two versus three or four agents and an overall survival advantage at 1 year in platinum versus non-platinum regimens. One of the major questions in this area has been the duration of treatment. Six versus four cycles of platinum-based doublet chemotherapy confer a longer progression-free survival, increased toxicity, and no overall survival advantage. The choice of the second agent depends on the physician and is usually decided based upon the toxicity profile of the agent. Cisplatin with paclitaxel, gemcitabine, or docetaxel and carboplatin with paclitaxel have all been shown to have similar efficacy. One of the largest trials to date has shown that, in contrast to lung adenocarcinoma, in SCC the combination of cisplatin and gemcitabine versus cisplatin and pemetrexed gives a longer median overall survival (10.8 months versus 9.4 months). Therefore, the use of pemetrexed in SCC is not recommended. Results from a meta-analysis show that when carboplatin is substituted for cisplatin the ORR is lower (24% versus 30%, odds ratio (OR) 1.37, 95% CI 1.16–1.61) and there is a non-significant trend towards shortened survival (median 8.4 versus 9.1 months, HR for death 1.07, 95% CI 0.99–1.15). The differences in the toxicity profiles of the two agents need to be taken into account when making treatment decisions.

The SQUIRE trial has recently shown that the addition of the anti-EGFR monoclonal antibody necitumumab to cisplatin and gemcitabine produced a modest but statistically significant overall improvement in survival (11.5 versus 9.9 months, HR 0.84, 95% CI 0.74–0.96, $P = 0.01$) and a 1 year survival of 48% versus 43% compared with cisplatin and gemcitabine alone. However, a retrospective analysis showed that the improvement was confined to patients with EGFR-expressing tumours (median overall survival 11.7 months versus 10.0 months, HR 0.79, 95% CI 0.69–0.92, $P = 0.002$); therefore, this regimen is licensed as a new first-line treatment option for advanced SCC expressing EGFR by IHC. Based on this trial, the FDA and EMA have approved the use of necitumumab with gemcitabine and cisplatin in the first-line treatment of advanced SCC. It has not been approved by the UK's National Institute for Health and Care Excellence (NICE) for cost-efficiency reasons.

The albumin-bound paclitaxel (nab-paclitaxel)–carboplatin (nab-PC) regimen has also been granted EMA and FDA approval based on the findings of a large phase III study on NSCLC in which it was shown to have a higher ORR and significantly less neurotoxicity than standard carboplatin–paclitaxel. Median overall survival was 12.1 months (95% CI 10.8–12.9 months) versus 11.2 months (95% CI 10.3–12.6 months) in the two groups, respectively. The results were more pronounced for the cohort of patients with squamous histology. The regime has not been approved by NICE.

If a patient is ineligible for treatment with cisplatin, a number of combinations can be considered, as follows. For patients older than 70 years with a performance status of 0–1 and selected patients with a performance status of 2, carboplatin-based chemotherapy is the preferred option. Patients with a performance status of 3–4 should not be offered chemotherapy in the absence of any EGFR mutations or ALK rearrangements.

Therapy following non-progression on first-line chemotherapy

No systemic therapy has demonstrated a survival advantage as maintenance so this is not recommended.

Second-line therapy for advanced SCC of the lung

Patients who progress on or after first-line chemotherapy should be offered second-line chemotherapy if they wish to have further treatment and their performance status is 0–2. Single-agent docetaxel is the treatment of choice in SCC, improving overall survival versus best supportive care. Pemetrexed is not indicated in SCC. Erlotinib is another option if patients are not fit for chemotherapy, or it can be given as a third-line treatment. Although licensed, erlotinib is no longer approved by NICE in this indication. In the second- and third-line setting docetaxel is associated with an increased progression-free survival but not overall survival compared with erlotinib. The addition of the vascular endothelial growth factor receptor-2 (VEGFR-2) inhibitor ramucirumab to docetaxel versus docetaxel and placebo showed an increased median overall survival (10.5 versus 9.1 months, HR 0.86, 95% CI 0.75–0.98) in all patients with NSCLC and a performance status of 0–2. Ramucirumab is therefore licensed in addition to docetaxel, but again is not approved by NICE due to cost-efficiency.

Learning points

- First-line treatment for advanced SCC of the lung in patients who have PD-L1 expression on at least 50% of their tumour cells should be with pembrolizumab in the absence of activating EGFR mutations or ALK translocations.

- In patients with tumours that have PD-L1 expression on <50% of their tumour cells, with EGFR- and ALK-negative disease and a performance status of 0–2, platinum-based doublet chemotherapy should be considered.

- Beyond progression there are currently a number of available treatment options licensed, including chemotherapy with docetaxel with/without ramucirumab, erlotinib, and anti-PD(L)-1 treatments in patients who have received first-line doublet chemotherapy and platinum-based doublet chemotherapy in patients who have had first-line pembrolizumab.

Further reading

Azzoli CG, Kris MG, Pfister DG. Cisplatin versus carboplatin for patients with metastatic non-small-cell lung cancer–an old rivalry renewed. J Natl Cancer Inst. 2007 Jun;**99**(11):828.

Brahmer J et al. Nivolumab versus docetaxel in advanced squamous-cell non-small-cell lung cancer. N Engl J Med. 2015 Jul;**373**(2):123–35.

Delbaldo C, Michiels S, Syz N, Soria JC, Le Chevalier T, Pignon JP. Benefits of adding a drug to a single-agent or a 2-agent chemotherapy regimen in advanced non-small-cell lung cancer: a meta-analysis. JAMA. 2004 Jul;**292**(4):470–84.

Des Guetz G, Uzzan B, Nicolas P, Valeyre D, Sebbane G, Morere JF. Comparison of the efficacy and safety of single-agent and doublet chemotherapy in advanced non-small cell lung cancer in the elderly: a meta-analysis. Crit Rev Oncol Hematol. 2012 Dec;**84**(3):340–9.

Garassino MC et al. Erlotinib versus docetaxel as second line treatment of patients with advanced non-small-cell lung cancer and wildtype EGFR tumours (TAILOR): a randomised controlled trial. Lancet Oncol. 2013 Sep;**14**(10):981–8.

Garon EB et al. Ramucirumab plus docetaxel versus placebo plus docetaxel for second-line treatment of stage IV non-small-cell lung cancer after disease progression on platinum-based therapy (REVEL): a multicentre, double-blind, randomised phase 3 trial. Lancet. 2014 Aug;**384**(9944):665–73.

Herbst RS et al. Pembrolizumab versus docetaxel for previously treated, PD-L1-positive, advanced non-small-cell lung cancer (KEYNOTE-010): a randomised controlled trial. Lancet. 2016 Apr;**387**(10027):1540.

Kawaguchi T et al. Randomized phase III trial of erlotinib versus docetaxel as second- or third-line therapy in patients with advanced nonsmall-cell lung cancer: Docetaxel and Erlotinib Lung Cancer Trial (DELTA). J Clin Oncol. 2014 Jun;**32**(18):1902–8.

Kerr KM et al. Second ESMO consensus conference on lung cancer: pathology and molecular biomarkers for non-small-cell lung cancer. Ann Oncol. 2014 Sep;**25**(9):1681–90.

Park JO et al. Phase III trial of two versus four additional cycles in patients who are nonprogressive after two cycles of platinum-based chemotherapy in non small-cell lung cancer. J Clin Oncol. 2007 Nov;**25**(33):5233–9.

Paz-Ares L, Socinski MA, Shahidi J, Hozak RR, Soldatenkova V, Thatcher N, Hirsch F. 1320_PR: subgroup analyses of patients with epidermal growth factor receptor (EGFR)-expressing tumors in SQUIRE: a randomized, multicenter, open-label, phase III study of gemcitabine cisplatin (GC) plus necitumumab (N) versus GC alone in the first-line treatment of patients (pts) with stage IV squamous non-small cell lung cancer (sq-NSCLC). J Thorac Oncol. 2016 Apr;**11**(4 Suppl):S153.

Pujol JL, Barlesi F, Daurès JP. Should chemotherapy combinations for advanced non-small cell lung cancer be platinum-based? A meta-analysis of phase III randomized trials. Lung Cancer. 2006 Mar;**51**(3):335–45.

Qi WX, Tang L, He AN, Shen Z, Lin F, Yao Y. Doublet versus single cytotoxic agent as first-line treatment for elderly patients with advanced non-small-cell lung cancer: a systematic review and meta-analysis. Lung. 2012 Oct;**190**(5):477–85.

Reck M et al. Pembrolizumab versus chemotherapy for PD-L1-positive non-small-cell lung cancer. N Engl J Med. 2016 Nov;**375**(19):1823.

Rekhtman N et al. Clarifying the spectrum of driver oncogene mutations in biomarker-verified squamous carcinoma of lung: lack of EGFR/KRAS and presence of PIK3CA/AKT1 mutations. Clin Cancer Res. 2012 Feb;**18**(4):1167–76.

Rittmeyer A et al. Atezolizumab versus docetaxel in patients with previously treated non-small-cell lung cancer (OAK): a phase 3, open-label, multicentre randomised controlled trial. Lancet. 2017 Jan;**389**(10066):255–65.

Rossi A et al. Six versus fewer planned cycles of first-line platinum-based chemotherapy for non-small-cell lung cancer: a systematic review and meta-analysis of individual patient data. Lancet Oncol. 2014 Oct;**15**(11):1254–62.

Scagliotti GV et al. Phase III study comparing cisplatin plus gemcitabine with cisplatin plus pemetrexed in chemotherapy-naive patients with advanced-stage non-small-cell lung cancer. J Clin Oncol. 2008 Jul;**26**(21):3543.

Schiller JH, Harrington D, Belani CP, Langer C, Sandler A, Krook J, Zhu J, Johnson DH; Eastern Cooperative Oncology Group. Comparison of four chemotherapy regimens for advanced non-small-cell lung cancer. N Engl J Med. 2002 Jan;**346**(2):92–8.

Shepherd FA et al. Prospective randomized trial of docetaxel versus best supportive care in patients with non-small-cell lung cancer previously treated with platinum-based chemotherapy. J Clin Oncol. 2000 May;**18**(10):2095–103.

Shepherd FA et al. Erlotinib in previously treated non-small-cell lung cancer. N Engl J Med. 2005 Jul;**353**(2):123–32.

Socinski MA et al. Weekly nab-paclitaxel in combination with carboplatin versus solvent-based paclitaxel plus carboplatin as first-line therapy in patients with advanced non-small-cell lung cancer: final results of a phase III trial. J Clin Oncol. 2012 Jun;**30**(17):2055–62.

Socinski M et al. CheckMate 026: A phase 3 trial of nivolumab vs investigator's choice (IC) of platinum-based doublet chemotherapy (PT-DC) as first-line therapy for stage iv/recurrent programmed death ligand 1 (PD-L1)-positive NSCLC. Ann Oncol. 2016 Oct;**27**(Suppl 6):LBA7_PR.

Syrigos KN et al. Prognostic and predictive factors in a randomized phase III trial comparing cisplatin-pemetrexed versus cisplatin-gemcitabine in advanced non-small-cell lung cancer. Ann Oncol. 2010 Mar;**21**(3):556.

Thatcher N et al. Necitumumab plus gemcitabine and cisplatin versus gemcitabine and cisplatin alone as first-line therapy in patients with stage IV squamous non-small-cell lung cancer (SQUIRE): an open-label, randomised, controlled phase 3 trial. Lancet Oncol. 2015 Jul;**16**(7):763–74.

Online resources

ESMO Clinical Practice Guidelines

◆ Novello S et al., Metastatic Non- Small- Cell Lung Cancer, http://www.esmo.org/Guidelines/ Lung-and-Chest-Tumours/Metastatic-Non-Small-Cell-Lung-Cancer

UpToDate

◆ Lilenbaum RC, Systemic therapy for the initial management of advanced non-small cell lung cancer without a driver mutation, https://www.uptodate.com/contents/systemic-therapy-for-advanced-non-small-cell-lung-cancer-with-an-activating-mutation-in-the-epidermal-growth-factor-receptor

◆ Gettinger S, Immunotherapy of non- small cell lung cancer with immune checkpoint inhibition, https://www.uptodate.com/contents/immunotherapy-of-non-small-cell-lung-cancer-with-immune-checkpoint-inhibition

◆ Sequist LV and Neal JW, Personalized, genotype- directed therapy for advanced non-small cell lung cancer, https://www.uptodate.com/contents/personalized-genotype-directed-therapy-for-advanced-non-small-cell-lung-cancer

Case 20

Non-resolving bilateral consolidation diagnosed as invasive mucinous adenocarcinoma with a lepidic predominant pattern (previously known as bronchoalveolar carcinoma) on biopsy

Adam Januszewski and Sanjay Popat

Case history

A 36 year old never smoker was referred to the respiratory physicians by her GP because of recurrent episodes of pneumonia. She described a cough productive of excessive volumes of white sputum. She did not complain of fevers or chills and her S_aO_2 was 95% on air. She had no other medical conditions and was not on any regular medications. Her World Health Organization (WHO) performance status was 0. A chest x-ray showed bilateral basal nodular opacification (Fig. 20.1). Blood tests showed her C-reactive protein (CRP) was 49 mg/L and her white cell count was 11.2×10^9/L. She had a short course of antibiotics. Given that she had multiple episodes of unresolving pneumonia and abnormal chest x-ray appearances she underwent a CT scan of the chest (Fig. 20.2a–d).

Questions

1. What does the CT scan show and what are the differential diagnoses?
2. What are the next steps in investigation and management?

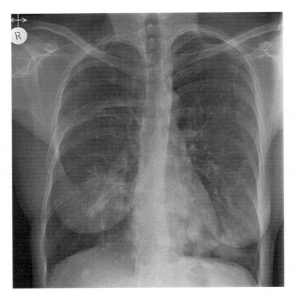

Fig. 20.1 Chest x-ray showing bilateral basal nodular opacification.

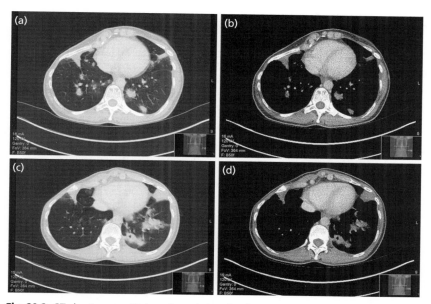

Fig. 20.2 CT chest scan with lung (a and c) and soft tissue (b and d) windows.

Answers

1. What does the CT scan show and what are the differential diagnoses?

The CT scan demonstrates bilateral multilobar ill-defined areas of consolidation. There are no discrete lesions or areas of invasion.

2. What are the next steps in investigation and management?

Given that the patient has failed to respond to numerous courses of antibiotics tissue sampling is required. This may include bronchoscopy for bronchial washings and biopsy of abnormal tissue.

Case history continued

The patient's symptoms failed to respond to antibiotics and, after a bronchoscopic lavage that demonstrated atypical cells (although not atypical enough to make a malignancy diagnosis), she proceeded to a CT-guided biopsy of an area that appeared more confluent/solid in the left lower lobe. The biopsy demonstrated a mucinous adenocarcinoma with a lepidic predominant pattern (previously known as bronchoalveolar carcinoma (BAC)). She received six cycles of platinum doublet chemotherapy with disease stability after six cycles as the best response. This was complicated by several admissions with non-neutropenic chest infections. The patient was slowly progressing 3 months later on chest x-ray and opted for ongoing watchful waiting prior to second-line systemic treatment.

Classification of lung adenocarcinomas (2015)

Recognizing the increased complexity of decision-making based upon histopathological assessment, a major reclassification of thoracic cancers generated more homogeneous subgroups that were designed to be better at predicting response and outcomes. Approximately 70% of lung cancers are diagnosed through small samples and therefore the 2015 WHO classification (Travis et al. 2015) also accounted for the use of small biopsy specimens as histological criteria for small biopsies had not been specified in previous WHO classifications. Terms that led to confusion and heterogeneous grouping as well as BAC and mixed subtype adenocarcinoma have been removed. Invasive adenocarcinomas have now also been reclassified according to their predominant pattern (Table 20.1).

Bronchoalveolar carcinoma reclassification

BAC was described in the 2004 WHO classification as a subtype of adenocarcinoma typified by its peripheral location, well-differentiated cytology, growth along intact alveolar septa, and potential to spread aerogenously or via the lymphatic system. In 2015 the WHO, in collaboration with the IASLC, American Thoracic Society

Table 20.1 International Association for the Study of Lung Cancer/American Thoracic Society/European Respiratory Society reclassification of lung adenocarcinomas

2004 Classification	Reclassification
Mixed subtype	Adenocarcinoma, describe identifiable patterns present (including micropapillary)
Acinar	
Papillary	
Solid	
Bronchoalveolar (non-mucinous) carcinoma	Adenocarcinoma with lepidic pattern (if pure, add: an invasive component cannot be excluded)
Bronchoalveolar (mucinous) carcinoma	Mucinous adenocarcinoma (describe patterns)
Fetal	Adenocarcinoma with fetal pattern
Mucinous (colloid)	Adenocarcinoma with colloid pattern
Signet ring	Adenocarcinoma with (describe pattern) and signet ring features
Clear cell	Adenocarcinoma with (describe pattern) and clear cell features
Not classified	Non-small-cell carcinoma, favour adenocarcinoma

Adapted from Travis, W.D. et al., (2011) International Association for the Study of Lung Cancer/American Thoracic Society/European Respiratory Society International Multidisciplinary Classification of Lung Adenocarcinoma. *Journal of Thoracic Oncology*, 6(2), pp.244–285 with permission from Elsevier.

(ATS), and the European Respiratory Society (ERS), led a major reclassification of BAC that included new subtypes to generate homogeneous entities to more accurately reflect the morphological, clinical, and biological subgroups (Travis et al. 2011).

Atypical adenomatous hyperplasia (AAH) is a term used to describe a preinvasive lesion that typically measures <5 mm. Adenocarcinoma in situ (AIS) describes lesions that are <3 cm and do not have any invasive components but typically have lepidic growth patterns (which describes the non-invasive growth along intact alveolar septa); most are non-mucinous. Both AAH and AIS have peripheral ground-glass characteristics on CT.

The new category of minimally invasive adenocarcinoma (MIA) describes lesions that are <3 cm, have an invasive component that is >5 mm, and are predominantly non-mucinous. These have ground-glass appearances with a more solid component on CT. The term invasive mucinous adenocarcinoma replaced the term mucinous BAC and describes the invasive spectrum of this classification with lepidic growth patterns and excessive mucin production (Table 20.2).

Disease spectrum and clinical presentation

AIS (previously BAC) with no invasive component has an extremely good prognosis with survival approaching 100% at 5 years. However, the range of more invasive subtypes adds complexity to this disease and their presentations are variable

Table 20.2 International Association for the Study of Lung Cancer/American Thoracic Society/European Respiratory Society reclassification of bronchoalveolar carcinomas

1. Adenocarcinoma in situ (AIS), which can be non-mucinous and rarely mucinous
2. Minimally invasive adenocarcinoma (MIA), which may be non-mucinous and rarely mucinous
3. Lepidic predominant adenocarcinoma (non-mucinous)
4. Adenocarcinoma, predominantly invasive with some non-mucinous lepidic component
5. Invasive mucinous adenocarcinoma (formerly mucinous BAC)

Adapted from Travis, W.D. et al., (2011) International Association for the Study of Lung Cancer/American Thoracic Society/European Respiratory Society International Multidisciplinary Classification of Lung Adenocarcinoma. *Journal of Thoracic Oncology*, 6(2), pp.244–285 with permission from Elsevier.

(Russell et al. 2011). Non-invasive AIS is often asymptomatic and identified incidentally. More invasive (minimally invasive through to invasive) disease appears as multiple peripheral nodules with variable solid phase components and ground-glass appearances (Breathnach et al. 1999).

Mucinous adenocarcinoma can present with diffuse bilateral disease that may resemble consolidative changes on imaging. Patients present with shortness of breath and cough with large volumes of white sputum (bronchorrhoea) and sometimes haemoptysis. This disease pattern is associated with a particularly poor prognosis. In advanced disease, metastases may be present at diagnosis and are similar to patterns of spread in NSCLC—bone, brain, and adrenal glands. In this case the patient presented with bilateral consolidative changes that failed to respond to antibacterial treatments, which would increase the suspicion of an invasive mucinous adenocarcinoma.

The aetiology of these tumours is not clearly understood. Patients are typically young and two-thirds are never or intermittent smokers. Although smoking may be a contributing factor, it is not the only one (Barsky et al. 1994) and other (yet unproven) postulated aetiologies include occupational exposure, scarring, and viral infections.

Imaging and diagnosis

Cross-sectional CT is required as part of the diagnosis and staging and to guide tissue collection. In the more aggressive mucinous adenocarcinomas it is difficult on CT to distinguish a malignant disease from bacterial infection. However, in less invasive, more nodular disease CT is important to characterize the nature of the pulmonary nodules and associated ground-glass opacities. The disease can progress slowly and therefore serial imaging may be required. PET scanning can also be unreliable in these tumours (particularly for the less invasive phenotypes) as they have a high false negative rate due to their slow rates of cell cycling.

Tissue diagnosis is required and access is dependent upon the disease subtype. Small peripheral lesions where the CT features are typical of an adenocarcinoma may be surgically resected for pathological assessment, although a percutaneous needle biopsy may be required if there is more extensive disease. Bronchoscopy washing can be performed, although, in order to make an accurate pathological diagnosis, sufficient tumour material is required to assess the presence (or lack of) invasive components of the disease. Furthermore, sufficient material is required for molecular analysis for other oncogenic drivers seen in non-smokers (e.g. EGFR mutations and ALK gene rearrangements) and therefore a transcutaneous biopsy is often required. Mucinous adenocarcinomas typically do not exhibit targetable oncogenic aberrations seen in other non-smokers with adenocarcinoma, although 80–100% of patients harbour a KRAS mutation—a somatic mutation that is not currently targetable with systemic therapy.

Treatment of advanced invasive mucinous adenocarcinoma

Locally invasive or operable multifocal adenocarcinoma should be treated as any other NSCLC with radical surgical resection. The treatment of advanced invasive mucinous adenocarcinoma is similar to that of other pulmonary adenocarcinomas in the absence of targetable oncogenic mutations. Although there are a few trials specifically investigating the effectiveness of chemotherapy in these patients (Scagliotti et al. 2005; West et al. 2005) most clinicians extrapolate data from large trials of patients with NSCLC to the invasive mucinous adenocarcinoma cohort. Standard of care in this case in the first-line setting with low PD-L1 expression (<50%) would therefore be platinum–pemetrexed doublet chemotherapy, and pembrolizumab monotherapy if PD-L1 expression ≥50%. However, response rates to chemotherapy are low and the outcomes generally poor.

Learning points

◆ The WHO classification of lung cancers (2015) creates a more comprehensive classification of pulmonary adenocarcinomas to generate homogeneous subtypes that more accurately reflect the morphological, clinical, and biological subgroups.

◆ Invasive mucinous adenocarcinoma (formerly mucinous BAC) is a rare tumour typically seen in young, female non-smokers.

◆ The disease can mimic a bilateral pneumonia presenting with shortness of breath and a cough productive of clear/white sputum with consolidative changes on imaging. In a patient with an unresolving pneumonic picture with the absence of fevers and raised inflammatory markers consider invasive mucinous adenocarcinoma.

◆ Definitive diagnosis should provide sufficient biological material to assess cellular and tissue architecture and therefore percutaneous biopsies are often necessary.

◆ Unlike many of the less invasive adenocarcinomas in the new classification, invasive mucinous adenocarcinoma has a particularly poor prognosis. Treatment is similar to that in other pulmonary adenocarcinomas, although response to first-line platinum doublet chemotherapy is often poor.

References

Barsky SH, Cameron R, Osann KE, Tomita D, Holmes EC. Rising incidence of bronchioloalveolar lung carcinoma and its unique clinicopathologic features. Cancer. 1994 Feb;**73**(4):1163–70.

Breathnach OS, Ishibe N, Williams J, Linnoila RI, Caporaso N, Johnson BE. Clinical features of patients with stage IIIB and IV bronchioloalveolar carcinoma of the lung. Cancer. 1999 Oct;**86**(7):1165–73.

Russell PA, Wainer Z, Wright GM, Daniels M, Conron M, Williams RA. Does lung adenocarcinoma subtype predict patient survival? A clinicopathologic study based on the new International Association for the Study of Lung Cancer/American Thoracic Society/European Respiratory Society international multidisciplinary lung adenocarcinoma classification. J Thorac Oncol. 2011 Sep;**6**(9):1496–504.

Scagliotti GV et al. A phase II study of paclitaxel in advanced bronchioloalveolar carcinoma (EORTC trial 08956). Lung Cancer. 2005 Oct;**50**(1):91–6.

Travis WD et al. International Association for the Study of Lung Cancer/American Thoracic Society/European Respiratory Society international multidisciplinary classification of lung adenocarcinoma. J Thorac Oncol. 2011 Feb;**6**(2):244–85.

Travis WD, Brambilla E, Burke AP, Marx A, Nicholson AG. WHO Classification of Tumours of the Lung, Pleura, Thymus and Heart. Lyon, France: International Agency for Research on Cancer; 2015.

West HL et al. Advanced bronchioloalveolar carcinoma: a phase II trial of paclitaxel by 96-hour infusion (SWOG 9714): a Southwest Oncology Group study. Ann Oncol. 2005 Jul;**16**(7):1076–80.

Further reading

Breathnach OS, Ishibe N, Williams J, Linnoila RI, Caporaso N, Johnson BE. Clinical features of patients with stage IIIB and IV bronchioloalveolar carcinoma of the lung. Cancer. 1999 Oct;**86**(7):1165–73.

Travis WD et al. International Association for the Study of Lung Cancer/American Thoracic Society/European Respiratory Society international multidisciplinary classification of lung adenocarcinoma.
J Thorac Oncol. 2011 Feb;**6**(2):244–85.

Case 21

Stage IIA adenocarcinoma of the lung in a never smoker undergoing adjuvant chemotherapy

Adam Januszewski and Sanjay Popat

Case history

A 45 year old never smoker was referred to the respiratory medicine service with an unresolving cough after a chest infection. Her chest x-ray demonstrated a right upper lobe opacity, which after cross-sectional imaging and bronchoscopic biopsy was found to be an adenocarcinoma of lung origin. Full staging (including PET-CT and MRI of the brain) identified no signs of nodal or distant disease. She had a WHO performance status of 0 and no other medical conditions. She proceeded to video-assisted thoracoscopic surgery (VATS) in which a right upper lobectomy with nodal resection of stations 2R, 4R, and 7 was carried out. Pathological assessment confirmed a 4.5 cm lung adenocarcinoma with no nodal involvement and clear margins (pT2bpN0M0R0)—stage IIA (eighth edition of the TNM classification for non-small-cell lung cancer). Molecular profiling was not performed.

Questions

1. According to the staging of this patient would this patient benefit from adjuvant treatments?

2. Other than stage what other considerations would you take into account when delivering adjuvant treatment?

3. The patient is aware that there are a lot of new developments for patients with lung cancer who have never smoked. She asks 'Why can I not receive some of these new treatments instead of chemotherapy?' What is your response?

Answers

1. According to the staging of this patient would this patient benefit from adjuvant treatments?

According to the eighth edition of the international TNM lung staging classification this patient has T2b disease, which equates to stage IIA. In the seventh edition of this classification this would have been classified as a T2a tumour and stage IB. A discussion with the patient about adjuvant cisplatin-based doublet chemotherapy would be indicated as this may reduce the risk of death. There is however no evidence that postoperative radiotherapy would be beneficial as she has clear resection margins (R0).

Adjuvant chemotherapy in NSCLC

Patients with stage I–III NSCLC have a significant chance of relapse and death from their disease despite complete resection of their tumour (40–70% depending on stage). Adjuvant systemic treatment aims to reduce the chance of relapse and subsequent death from their disease and is offered to patients with resected stage II and IIIA NSCLC. The evidence for this is borne out by several large studies and evaluated in the LACE (Lung Adjuvant Cisplatin Evaluation) meta-analysis. This meta-analysis combined individual data from 4584 patients with a median follow-up of 5.2 years from the five largest adjuvant trials in lung cancer and demonstrated a survival benefit (Pignon et al. 2008). The use of adjuvant cisplatin doublet chemotherapy demonstrated a 5.3% benefit in overall survival and a 5.2% benefit in progression-free survival at 5 years compared with no chemotherapy (HR for death 0.83, 95% CI 0.82–0.96), with an absolute survival benefit at 5 years increasing with greater resected stage.

The adjuvant treatment of stage IB disease as described by the seventh edition of the UICC TNM classification (stage IIA in the eighth edition) with chemotherapy remains controversial. The CALGB 9633 study of adjuvant carboplatin–paclitaxel first suggested a benefit of adjuvant chemotherapy in patients with large stage IB tumours. In an unplanned analysis a statistically significant improvement in overall survival in stage IB disease when the tumour was ≥4 cm was demonstrated (Strauss et al. 2008). The LACE meta-analysis of primary trials investigating the benefit of adjuvant chemotherapy or not after surgery demonstrated a trend towards improved survival in patients with stage IB disease, based on a small sample size. In the JBR-10 randomized trial (which formed part of the LACE meta-analysis; Butts et al. 2010) the updated long-term follow-up (median 9.2 years) demonstrated that while patients with stage IB disease did not benefit from chemotherapy per se, when accounting for tumour size, those with tumours ≥4 cm derived a clinically meaningful survival benefit with adjuvant chemotherapy (HR 0.66, 95% CI 0.39–1.14). This is one of the reasons that the UICC T descriptor now reclassifies tumours >4 cm as T2b.

2. Other than stage what other considerations would you take into account when delivering adjuvant treatment?

The benefit of adjuvant chemotherapy is seen in patients with a better performance status. Comorbidities, in particular cardiovascular disease, may direct the cisplatin partner; however, typically four cycles of cisplatin and vinorelbine could be offered between 6 and 8 weeks after surgery.

Risk stratification and patient selection

TNM classification and disease stage remain the strongest predictors of benefit from adjuvant chemotherapy, which in fact is detrimental to those patients with stage IA disease. In patients with lower pathological stages whose benefit from adjuvant chemotherapy is less, patient selection is important. In a large 'real-life' evaluation of 30 day mortality in patients across England treated with 'curative' chemotherapy in lung cancer there was a mortality rate of 3% (Wallington et al. 2016). Therefore, careful evaluation of high-risk disease (such as lymphovascular invasion, tumour size and differentiation, and extent of visceral pleural involvement) as well as patients at risk of adverse events from chemotherapy is needed. Patients with a lower WHO performance status benefit more from adjuvant chemotherapy while those with a WHO performance status of 2 do not benefit. In a subgroup analysis of the JBR-10 trial by Pepe et al. (2007) older patients appeared to benefit similarly to younger patients although they received fewer total doses of cisplatin. As part of patient evaluation it is important to consider their comorbidities (in particular cardiovascular disease) as this is the highest cause of non-cancer-related mortality when evaluated up to 6 months during follow-up. Furthermore, in the Ontario Cancer Registry Study there was a detrimental effect of adjuvant chemotherapy in those patients with a higher number of comorbidities (Booth et al. 2013).

3. The patient is aware that there are a lot of new developments for patients with lung cancer who have never smoked. She asks 'Why can I not receive some of these new treatments instead of chemotherapy?' What is your response?

Trials continue in evaluating the use of targeted agents in patients with oncogenic mutant lung cancers. Currently, however, there is no trial evidence that the use of EGFR- or ALK-directed therapies in the adjuvant setting improves overall survival.

What chemotherapy regimen, how much, and when?

Cisplatin-based chemotherapies have been most investigated in the adjuvant setting. The LACE meta-analysis failed to identify an optimal regimen although cisplatin–vinorelbine appeared marginally better than other combinations in this study

(Pignon et al. 2008). The E1505 trial, although not designed to detect differences between cisplatin doublets, did not detect variations in overall survival between regimens. However, there were differences in the toxicity profiles (Wakelee et al. 2016); therefore, this should be taken into consideration when choosing the cisplatin partner. Four cycles of doublet chemotherapy are sufficient to derive benefit when the cumulative dose is >300 mg/m^2. This is most likely to be achieved in the cisplatin–vinorelbine doublet than in other combinations, which lends further weight to its use (Pignon et al. 2008).

Cisplatin is the platinum partner of choice as it has been tested in adjuvant trials. The differences between carboplatin and cisplatin have not been systematically evaluated in this setting. Cisplatin induces thrombosis and platelet aggregation, and its administration requires significant intravenous hydration that can be difficult to manage with impaired cardiac function. Therefore, consideration of the platinum agent is important and some oncologists use carboplatin instead for patients in whom there is concern regarding cardiac/renal function or issues with neuropathy/hearing loss or emetogenicity. However, its use should be with the caveat that its efficacy is not proven and it carries the potential risk of increased myelosuppression.

Adjuvant chemotherapy typically begins within 8 weeks of surgery should the patient have recovered sufficiently to tolerate systemic chemotherapy. Although oncologists aim to deliver the chemotherapy 6–8 weeks after surgery, sometimes it is not possible and even delayed adjuvant chemotherapy (up to 4 months) improves overall outcome compared with those who have surgery alone (Salazar et al. 2017). Although postoperative radiotherapy is not routine, it is delivered in some circumstances such as positive resection margins (R1); in these cases this would follow the completion of adjuvant chemotherapy, sequentially.

Molecular analysis and targeted treatments in the adjuvant setting

Evidence of oncogenic molecular drivers in patients with lung cancer that are never smokers continues to grow. The use of targeted agents directed at EGFR activating mutations, ALK–echinoderm microtubule-associated protein-like-4 (EML4) gene rearrangements, and ROS-1 fusions in the advanced setting has a good evidence base and is making clinically meaningful improvements in progression-free survival. Overall survival has been more difficult to demonstrate in these populations because of cross-over treatments in trials and because patients with these tumours have a different clinical course from smokers. Logic may dictate that if a resected tumour has a targetable oncogenic mutation then the use of a targeted agent in the adjuvant rather than cytotoxic chemotherapy may provide clinical benefit to these patients. Studies evaluating the use of EGFR targeting agents in the adjuvant setting (in both the selected and unselected population—RADIANT and BR19 trials), although demonstrating a trend towards improved progression-free survival, failed to show an improvement in overall survival (Goss et al. 2013; Kelly et al. 2015) and have identified a higher rate of brain metastases on relapse. Trials in this setting are ongoing. The standard of care for adjuvant treatment in never smokers therefore remains the use of chemotherapy (Vansteenkiste et al. 2016). On the basis that molecular testing and predictive biomarkers do not direct the use of adjuvant therapies molecular testing of targetable oncogenic drivers of resection specimens is not routinely recommended, although it can be considered on an individual basis for optimal laboratory sample workflow purposes. Molecular characterization of the tumour can aid future treatment in the event of disease relapse, although this can be performed on archived surgical specimens at the time of relapse.

Immunotherapy in the adjuvant setting

Using the immune system to target lung cancer has become a treatment modality in both the first- and second-line settings in patients with advanced disease. Impressive outcomes have been demonstrated that supersede conventional chemotherapy regimens and have favourable toxicity profiles. However, determining the patient cohorts that derive benefit has been more difficult, although there is evidence that mutational burden (induced by smoking) is a good surrogate predictive biomarker for response to immune checkpoint inhibitors. Its use in the adjuvant setting is being tested, although in the case of a never smoker one may question the clinical efficacy in these patients. In the largest ever randomized phase III trial to date in the adjuvant setting, patients with resected NSCLC were given a vaccine directed against the MAGE-A3 tumour antigen. However, this has failed to demonstrate an improvement in overall survival (Groen et al. 2016). There are a number of trials of immune checkpoint inhibitors underway targeting different receptors of the immune synapse in the adjuvant setting.

Learning points

♦ Adjuvant platinum doublet chemotherapy in patients with resected stage IIA–IIIA (eighth edition TNM staging) NSCLC improves 5 year overall survival.

♦ Patients with node-negative large tumours ($\geq$4 cm) may benefit from adjuvant chemotherapy but patient selection is important.

♦ Four cycles of chemotherapy with a total dose >300 mg/m^2 of cisplatin should be offered to patients up to 4 months after resection.

♦ Performance status and comorbidities should be taken into account when offering patients adjuvant chemotherapy and can dictate the most suitable platinum doublet.

♦ Trials are ongoing investigating the use of targeted agents and immunotherapy in the adjuvant setting, although currently there is no evidence for their use.

References

Booth CM, Shepherd FA, Peng Y, Darling G, Li G, Kong W, Biagi JJ, Mackillop WJ. Time to adjuvant chemotherapy and survival in non-small cell lung cancer: a population-based study. Cancer. 2013 Mar;**119**(6):1243–50.

Butts CA et al. Randomized phase III trial of vinorelbine plus cisplatin compared with observation in completely resected stage IB and II non-small-cell lung cancer: updated survival analysis of JBR-10. J Clin Oncol. 2010 Jan;**28**(1):29–34.

Goss GD et al. Gefitinib versus placebo in completely resected non-small-cell lung cancer: results of the NCIC CTG BR19 study. J Clin Oncol. 2013 Sep;**31**(27):3320–6.

Groen HJM et al. Randomized phase III study of adjuvant immunotherapy with or without low-molecular weight heparin in completely resected non-small cell lung cancer patients. J Clin Oncol. 2016;**34**(15 Suppl):8506–6.

Kelly K et al. Adjuvant erlotinib versus placebo in patients with stage IB-IIIA non-small-cell lung cancer (RADIANT): a randomized, double-blind, phase III trial. J Clin Oncol. 2015 Dec;**33**(34):4007–14.

Pepe C et al. Adjuvant vinorelbine and cisplatin in elderly patients: National Cancer Institute of Canada and Intergroup Study JBR.10. J Clin Oncol. 2007 Apr;**25**(12):1553–61.

Pignon JP et al. Lung adjuvant cisplatin evaluation: a pooled analysis by the LACE Collaborative Group. J Clin Oncol. 2008 Jul;**26**(21):3552–9.

Salazar MC et al. Association of delayed adjuvant chemotherapy with survival after lung cancer surgery. JAMA Oncol. 2017 May;**3**(5):610–19.

Strauss GM et al. Adjuvant paclitaxel plus carboplatin compared with observation in stage IB non-small-cell lung cancer: CALGB 9633 with the Cancer and Leukemia Group B, Radiation Therapy Oncology Group, and North Central Cancer Treatment Group Study Groups. J Clin Oncol. 2008 Nov;**26**(31):5043–51.

Vansteenkiste J et al. 2nd ESMO Consensus Conference on Lung Cancer: early-stage non-small-cell lung cancer consensus on diagnosis, treatment and follow-up. Ann Oncol. 2014 Aug;**25**(8):1462–74.

Wakelee HA et al. ECOG-ACRIN. Adjuvant chemotherapy with or without bevacizumab in patients with resected non-small-cell lung cancer (E1505): an open-label, multicentre, randomised, phase 3 trial. Lancet Oncol. 2017 Dec;**18**(12):1610–23.

Wallington M et al. 30-day mortality after systemic anticancer treatment for breast and lung cancer in England: a population-based, observational study. Lancet Oncol. 2016 Sep;**17**(9):1203–16.

Further reading

LACE meta-analysis: Pignon JP et al. Lung adjuvant cisplatin evaluation: a pooled analysis by the LACE Collaborative Group. J Clin Oncol. 2008 Jul;**26**(21):3552–9.

ESMO guidelines for the management of early stage non-small-cell lung cancer: Vansteenkiste J et al. 2nd ESMO Consensus Conference on Lung Cancer: early-stage non-small-cell lung cancer consensus on diagnosis, treatment and follow-up. Ann Oncol. 2014 Aug;**25**(8):1462–74.

Case 22

Malignant pleural mesothelioma

Spyros Gennatas and Sanjay Popat

Case history

A 57 year old white female who was a widow presented to her GP with a 2 month history of persistent, irritating, dry cough. She had had no symptoms suggestive of an upper or lower respiratory tract infection prior to that. She was otherwise in good health apart from experiencing generalized fatigue, which was not affecting her activities of daily living. She was a retired biology teacher and a never smoker. She had no past medical history of any other conditions and was not on any regular medications. Her mother was still alive and in reasonably good health but her father had died of an 'eye cancer' when he was 60. Clinical examination was unremarkable. Oxygen saturation was 97% on room air.

A set of routine blood tests, including a full blood count and biochemistry (urea and electrolytes, creatinine, liver function tests, and CRP), was unremarkable. Chest x-ray showed irregular pleural thickening.

Questions

1. What is the investigation of choice at this stage?
2. What is the most appropriate next step?
3. Given these findings is there any extra history you would like to take?
4. How would you treat this patient?
5. What treatment options are available on relapse?
6. What is the significance of the patient's family history and how does it need to be addressed?

Answers

1. What is the investigation of choice at this stage?

A contrast-enhanced CT scan of the chest and upper abdomen is the investigation of choice at this stage.

Case history continued

The CT scan was consistent with a T4M0 mesothelioma (stage IV) as per the International Mesothelioma Interest Group (IMIG)/UICC staging system.

2. What is the most appropriate next step?

Tissue diagnosis is essential to establish a diagnosis. The preferred method is via thoracoscopy, whether via pleuroscopy or VATS. Multiple biopsies from malignant- and normal-looking tissue are recommended given the diagnostic difficulty and the medicolegal significance of establishing the diagnosis.

Case history continued

In this case a VATS biopsy revealed an epithelioid mesothelioma via IHC.

3. Given these findings is there any extra history you would like to take?

A detailed occupational history is essential: specifically, whether either she or her deceased husband had any exposure to asbestos.

4. How would you treat this patient?

The recommended treatment for malignant pleural mesothelioma (MPM) is combination chemotherapy with cisplatin plus pemetrexed doublet. The role of cytoreductive surgery for MPM is currently debatable.

Primary systemic therapy for unresectable malignant pleural mesothelioma

First-line chemotherapy for MPM has been shown to improve survival. Doublet chemotherapy with cisplatin and pemetrexed has become the standard of care world-wide based on a phase III trial that showed an overall survival advantage with the addition of pemetrexed to cisplatin alone. Pemetrexed should always be given with prophylactic folic acid and vitamin B12. Carboplatin is a reasonable alternative to cisplatin in more frail patients as it less toxic and better tolerated. The large phase III MAPS trial in France showed the addition of bevacizumab to six cycles of cisplatin and pemetrexed with 3 weekly maintenance thereafter resulted in progression-free and overall survival benefit over chemotherapy alone in patients with MPM with a performance status of 0–1 and no contraindications to bevacizumab treatment. Based on this study this is rapidly becoming the standard of care in France, although the regime is currently unlicensed.

5. What treatment options are available on relapse?

There is currently no standard second-line treatment for MPM, although platinum–pemetrexed rechallenge, vinorelbine, and gemcitabine are commonly used. It is therefore recommended that patients who progress following fist-line chemotherapy are enrolled into clinical trials. Immune checkpoint inhibitors, such as the anti-PD-1 antibody pembrolizumab, are currently showing promising results in early clinical trials in this patient cohort.

Postprogression systemic therapy for malignant pleural mesothelioma

There is currently no consensus on second-line treatment for patients who have progressed/relapsed following first-line chemotherapy. Platinum–pemetrexed rechallenge is commonly used if the treatment-free interval is long (usually >6 months). Single-agent chemotherapy with vinorelbine or gemcitabine has shown activity, but there have been no randomized trials of these agents in this setting. Entry into ongoing clinical trials is therefore recommended when available and the patient's condition allows.

The role of immunotherapy in malignant pleural mesothelioma

As in many other solid tumours the treatment of MPM with immune checkpoint inhibitors has offered very promising results so far. A mesothelioma-specific cohort of the KEYNOTE-028 trial identified a response rate of 20% for patients treated with the anti-PD-1 antibody pembrolizumab. The overall disease control rate was 81%. The overall survival was a median of 18 months. PD-L1 expression in $\geq$1% of the tumour cells by IHC was a key eligibility criterion for entry into the study. Similarly in the JAVELIN phase Ib trial of 53 patients with MPM, following platinum-based first-line chemotherapy and no selection based on PD-L1 status, five patients exhibited a partial response and 25 had stable disease giving an overall disease control rate of 56.6%.

6. What is the significance of the patient's family history and how does it need to be addressed?

Mesothelioma has been recently been identified as one of a few tumours associated with the BAP1 tumour predisposition syndrome (BAP1-TPDS). As with all malignancies, especially those that present at an early age or in the absence of established risk factors, a detailed personal and family history of any malignancy needs to be obtained. In this case the history of the father, who died of an 'eye cancer', is highly suggestive of a uveal melanoma, which is one of the cancers associated with this syndrome.

The role of BAP1 in family history-taking of patients with MPM

BAP1-TPDS is a diagnosis based on molecular genetic testing that identifies a heterozygous germline pathogenic variant in BAP1. Its prevalence is unknown but a review in 2015 identified 57 families with 174 individuals with BAP1-TPDS in the existing literature. It is inherited in an autosomal dominant manner and is linked with an increased risk of developing atypical Spitz tumours and a number of cancers including uveal melanoma (commonest), mesothelioma, cutaneous melanoma, clear cell renal cell carcinoma, and basal cell carcinoma among others. An affected individual can develop many of these primary tumours at a median age of onset that is younger than the rest of the population who develop these malignancies. Mesothelioma is the second commonest cancer associated with BAP1-TPDS and is identified in 22% of cases. The median age of onset for mesothelioma in this group is younger than that expected for sporadic mesothelioma at 55–58 years. There are disproportionately more cases of peritoneal mesothelioma versus MPM in this group with the majority of peritoneal cases encountered in women, in contrast to the general population. Whereas other malignancies in this syndrome behave more aggressively than in the general population patients with mesothelioma in many cases follow a more indolent course. In the presence of pathogenic BAP1 variants exposure to asbestos significantly increases the risk of developing mesothelioma.

When an individual has had two or more of the above malignancies or has one malignancy and a first- or second-degree relative who has one of these tumours, BAP1-TPDS needs to be considered and a referral for genetic counselling needs to be made.

Genetic counselling referral

BAP1-TPDS is an autosomal dominant condition. Most individuals diagnosed have an affected parent and the incidence of de novo pathogenic BAP1 variants remains unknown. Although the expected chance of a child inheriting the syndrome from an affected individual is 50% the actual proportion varies significantly between families, presumably because of incomplete penetrance, as does the type of tumours that develop in members of the same family. Molecular genetic testing is recommended for all first- and second-degree relatives of diagnosed patients to facilitate early screening and/or preventative measures.

Learning points

- MPM is treated with doublet chemotherapy with cisplatin/carboplatin and pemetrexed. The addition of bevacizumab improves survival when combined with cisplatin–pemetrexed.

- The emergence of immune checkpoint inhibitors, in particular anti-PD-1/PD-L1 antibodies, is very promising and is currently under evaluation in ongoing clinical trials.

- BAP1-TPDS is a rare condition, with affected individuals having an increased predisposition to a number of malignancies, including mesothelioma.

- Genetic counselling of affected individuals and molecular gene testing of first- and second-degree relatives is recommended.

Further reading

Alley EW, Molife LR, Santoro A, Beckey K, Yuan S, Cheng JD, Piperdi B, Schellens JHM. Clinical safety and efficacy of pembrolizumab (MK-3475) in patients with malignant pleural mesothelioma: preliminary results from KEYNOTE-028. Cancer Res. 2015 Aug;**75**(15 Suppl):CT103.

Armato SG III, Labby ZE, Coolen J, Klabatsa A, Feigen M, Persigehl T, Gill RR. Imaging in pleural mesothelioma: a review of the 11th International Conference of the International Mesothelioma Interest Group. Lung Cancer. 2013 Nov;**82**(2):190–6.

Castagneto B et al. Phase II study of pemetrexed in combination with carboplatin in patients with malignant pleural mesothelioma (MPM). Ann Oncol. 2008 Feb;**19**(2):370–3.

Ceresoli GL et al. Phase II study of pemetrexed plus carboplatin in malignant pleural mesothelioma. J Clin Oncol. 2006 Mar;**24**(9):1443–8.

Greillier L, Cavailles A, Fraticelli A, Scherpereel A, Barlesi F, Tassi G, Thomas P, Astoul P. Accuracy of pleural biopsy using thoracoscopy for the diagnosis of histologic subtype in patients with malignant pleural mesothelioma. Cancer. 2007 Nov;**110**(10):2248–52.

Hassan R et al. Avelumab (MSB0010718C; anti-PD-L1) in patients with advanced unresectable mesothelioma from the JAVELIN solid tumor phase Ib trial: Safety, clinical activity, and PD-L1 expression. J Clin Oncol. 2016;**34**(15 Suppl):8503.

Maskell NA, Gleeson FV, Davies RJ. Standard pleural biopsy versus CT-guided cutting-needle biopsy for diagnosis of malignant disease in pleural effusions: a randomised controlled trial. Lancet. 2003 Apr;**361**(9366):1326–30.

Muers MF et al. Active symptom control with or without chemotherapy in the treatment of patients with malignant pleural mesothelioma (MS01): a multicentre randomised trial. Lancet. 2008 May;**371**(9625):1685–94.

Pilarski R, Rai K, Cebulla C, Abdel-Rahman M. BAP1 tumor predisposition syndrome. 2016 Oct 13. In: Pagon RA, Adam MP, Ardinger HH, et al, editors. GeneReviews® [Internet]. Seattle (WA): University of Washington, Seattle; 1993–2017. Available at https://www.ncbi.nlm.nih.gov/books/NBK390611/

Rusch VW. A proposed new international TNM staging system for malignant pleural mesothelioma. From the International Mesothelioma Interest Group. Chest. 1995 Oct;**108**(4):1122–8.

Santoro A et al. Pemetrexed plus cisplatin or pemetrexed plus carboplatin for chemonaïve patients with malignant pleural mesothelioma: results of the International Expanded Access Program. J Thorac Oncol. 2008 Jul;**3**(7):756–63.

Stebbing J et al. The efficacy and safety of weekly vinorelbine in relapsed malignant pleural mesothelioma. Lung Cancer. 2009 Jan;**63**(1):94–7.

Vogelzang NJ et al. Phase III study of pemetrexed in combination with cisplatin versus cisplatin alone in patients with malignant pleural mesothelioma. J Clin Oncol. 2003 Jul;**21**(14):2636.

Zalcman G et al. Bevacizumab for newly diagnosed pleural mesothelioma in the Mesothelioma Avastin Cisplatin Pemetrexed Study (MAPS): a randomised, controlled, open-label, phase 3 trial. Lancet. 2016 Apr;**387**(10026):1405–14.

Zauderer MG, Kass SL, Woo K, Sima CS, Ginsberg MS, Krug LM. Vinorelbine and gemcitabine as second- or third-line therapy for malignant pleural mesothelioma. Lung Cancer. 2014 Jun;**84**(3):271–4.

Online resources

ESMO Clinical Practice Guidelines

◆ Bass P et al., Malignant Pleural Mesothelioma, http://www.esmo.org/Guidelines/Lung-and-Chest-Tumours/Malignant-Pleural-Mesothelioma

National Cancer Institute

◆ Malignant Mesothelioma Treatment (PDQ®)–Health Professional Version, https://www.cancer.gov/types/mesothelioma/hp/mesothelioma-treatment-pdq

UpToDate

◆ Tsao AS and Vogelzang N, Systemic treatment for unresectable malignant pleural mesothelioma, https://www.uptodate.com/contents/systemic-treatment-for-unresectable-malignant-pleural-mesothelioma

Case 23

Lung carcinoid tumour

Spyros Gennatas and Sanjay Popat

Case history

A 45 year old male presented to his GP with a sore throat and general malaise for a period of 4 weeks. He was otherwise well with no other symptoms or significant past medical history. He did not have a family history of any serious medical conditions. He was not on any regular medications and was a never smoker. He had been extremely busy and had put off seeing his GP for a while. The duration of his symptoms and his wife's concerns motivated him to do so.

On examination he looked well although a bit stressed. His observations were all unremarkable and his oxygen saturation was 96% on room air. Examination of his chest revealed reduced breath sounds and associated dullness on percussion at the left upper chest.

Questions

1. What would you do next to investigate the cause of this male's signs and symptoms?
2. What imaging investigations would you perform next?
3. What would you do to obtain a diagnosis?
4. Are there any other investigations that you need to perform at this stage?
5. How would you treat this patient?

Answers

1. What would you do next to investigate the cause of this male's signs and symptoms?

Given the symptoms and worrying signs, the investigation of choice at this stage would be a chest x-ray, which can be done the same day and guide further investigations if needed.

Case history continued

A chest x-ray performed at the nearest hospital revealed a left upper lobe mass.

2. What imaging investigations would you perform next?

A contrast-enhanced CT scan of the chest and upper abdomen should be performed next.

Case history continued

The CT scan revealed a 5.5 cm left upper lobe mass consistent with malignancy. There was also ipsilateral and contralateral mediastinal lymph node involvement with multiple distant metastases identified in the bones. The stage of the disease was therefore T3N3M1b (stage IVB) according to UICC.

3. What would you do to obtain a diagnosis?

Bronchoscopy and biopsy of the mass is required.

Case history continued

Bronchoscopy and biopsy of the mass revealed an atypical carcinoid tumour (8 mitoses per mm^2) that was TTF-1 and chromogranin positive.

4. Are there any other investigations that you need to perform at this stage?

Around 80% of typical and 60% of atypical bronchial neuroendocrine tumours (NETs) express somatostatin receptors on IHC. They can therefore be imaged using an octreotide scan (^{111}In-pentetreotide; octreoscan). Octreotide is a radiolabelled somatostatin analogue and allows visualization of metastatic disease across the body. Baseline use of an octreotide scan is recommended in patients with advanced disease, as a positive scan is highly predictive of response to treatment with somatostatin analogues such as octreotide or lanreotide.

An FDA-licensed alternative is the use of PET with the tracer ^{68}Ga-DOTATATE, which has been shown to be more sensitive in the detection of small lesions.

Case history continued

In this case an octreotide scan was performed. All sites of disease visualized on CT were positive. No additional disease sites were revealed.

5. How would you treat this patient?

The patient should be commenced on treatment with octreotide.

Systemic therapy for carcinoid tumours of the lung

Lung NETs can be classified into four subtypes: well-differentiated, low-grade typical carcinoids (2% of primary lung cancers); well-differentiated, intermediate-grade atypical carcinoids (<1%); poorly differentiated, high-grade large-cell neuroendocrine carcinomas (3%); and poorly differentiated, high-grade small-cell lung cancers (20%). The WHO refers to typical and atypical carcinoid tumours simply as carcinoid tumours. These are rare tumours characterized by neuroendocrine differentiation and are commonly low-grade, indolent tumours compared with other lung neoplasms. Given their rarity there is very little evidence from prospective clinical trials to guide the management of advanced disease. A multidisciplinary approach to the care of such patients is therefore essential. Data from commoner NETs, such as those of the gastrointestinal tract, are often used. Surgery is an option for patients whose disease can be completely excised, including those with stage III disease and stage IV disease if completely resectable.

Systemic chemotherapy currently is recommended when other treatment options are not available. Commonly used regimens include cisplatin–etoposide and temozolomide monotherapy.

Somatostatin analogues

Although evidence for use of these drugs is based on experience from gastrointestinal NETs, patients whose tumours are somatostatin receptor positive based on their diagnostic imaging are commonly treated with the somatostatin analogues octreotide or lanreotide as first line. There are currently no clinical trial data on the use of these drugs in bronchial NETs.

Molecular targeted therapy for carcinoid tumours of the lung

The RADIANT-4 trial—a randomized, placebo-controlled, phase III study—evaluated the efficacy of the mechanistic target of rapamycin kinase (mTOR) inhibitor everolimus in 302 patients with bronchial or gastrointestinal NETs that were somatostatin receptor negative on somatostatin receptor scintigraphy. Progression-free survival was prolonged versus placebo (11.0 and 3.9 months, respectively; HR 0.48, 95% CI 0.35–0.67). The disease control rate was 81% versus 64% in patients having everolimus and placebo, respectively. In the lung NET subpopulation a post hoc subgroup analysis showed a progression-free survival for everolimus of 9.2 versus 3.6 months with placebo (HR 0.50, 95% CI 0.28–0.88). The FDA and EMA have approved everolimus for the treatment of adults with progressive, well-differentiated, non-functional lung or gastrointestinal NETs with unresectable, locally advanced or metastatic disease.

Locoregional therapies

Radiofrequency ablation of the tumour, whether in the lung or liver, and cryoablation, hepatic artery embolization, or chemoembolization with drugs such as doxorubicin (transarterial chemoembolization) of liver lesions are often used in conjunction with or instead of surgery.

Peptide receptor radiotargeted/radionuclide therapy

NETs that express subtype 2 somatostatin receptors can be identified by ^{111}In-labelled somatostatin analogue scintigraphy or ^{68}Ga-labelled somatostatin analogue PET scans, which constitute predictors of response. Peptide receptor radiotargeted/radionuclide therapy can be used to treat metastatic disease using ^{90}Y-DOTA octreotide or ^{177}Lu-DOTA octreotide. ^{177}Lu-DOTA octreotate (DOTATATE), which is a combination of the beta-emitting lutetium coupled with octreotate, has also shown promising results in small studies and proven benefit in a randomized trial in midgut carcinoid tumours.

Learning points

◆ Patients with advanced stage lung NETs with tumours that are somatostatin receptor positive can be treated with somatostatin analogues such as octreotide or lanreotide as first line.

◆ For somatostatin-receptor-negative tumours treatment with everolimus is an appropriate option.

◆ Cisplatin or temozolomide-based chemotherapy are reasonable options when the above treatments are not available.

◆ Peptide receptor radiotargeted/radionuclide therapy is an option for patients with subtype 2 somatostatin-expressing tumours.

Further reading

Caplin ME et al. Pulmonary neuroendocrine (carcinoid) tumors: European Neuroendocrine Tumor Society expert consensus and recommendations for best practice for typical and atypical pulmonary carcinoid. Ann Oncol. 2015 Aug;**26**(8):1604–20.

Crona J, Fanola I, Lindholm DP, Antonodimitrakis P, Öberg K, Eriksson B, Granberg D. Effect of temozolomide in patients with metastatic bronchial carcinoids. Neuroendocrinology. 2013;**98**(2):151.

Granberg D, Eriksson B, Wilander E, Grimfjärd P, Fjällskog ML, Oberg K, Skogseid B. Experience in treatment of metastatic pulmonary carcinoid tumors. Ann Oncol. 2001 Oct;**12**(10):1383.

Hendifar AE, Marchevsky AM, Tuli R. Neuroendocrine tumors of the lung: current challenges and advances in the diagnosis and management of well-differentiated disease. J Thorac Oncol. 2016 Mar;**12**(3):425–36.

Imhof A et al. Response, survival, and long-term toxicity after therapy with the radiolabeled somatostatin analogue [90Y-DOTA]-TOC in metastasized neuroendocrine cancers. J Clin Oncol. 2011 Jun;**29**(17):2416–23.

Jermendy G, Kónya A, Kárpáti P. Hepatic artery embolisation—new approach for treatment of malignant carcinoid syndrome. Dtsch Z Verdau Stoffwechselkr. 1986;**46**:130.

Kwekkeboom DJ, de Herder WW, Kam BL, van Eijck CH, van Essen M, Kooij PP, Feelders RA, van Aken MO, Krenning EP. Treatment with the radiolabeled somatostatin analog [177Lu-DOTA0,Tyr3]octreotate: toxicity, efficacy, and survival. J Clin Oncol. 2008 May;**26**(13):2124–30.

Mojtahedi A, Thamake S, Tworowska I, Ranganathan D, Delpassand ES. The value of (68)Ga-DOTATATE PET/CT in diagnosis and management of neuroendocrine tumors compared to current FDA approved imaging modalities: a review of literature. Am J Nucl Med Mol Imaging. 2014 Aug;**4**(5):426–34.

National Comprehensive Cancer Network. Neuroendocrine Tumors. National Comprehensive Cancer Network Clinical Practice Guidelines in Oncology, Version 1.2017, published 21 February 2017. Fort Washington, PA: National Comprehensive Cancer Network. Available at https://www.nccn.org/professionals/physician_gls/PDF/neuroendocrine.pdf

National Comprehensive Cancer Network. Small Cell Lung Cancer. National Comprehensive Cancer Network Clinical Practice Guidelines in Oncology, Version 3.2017, published 23 February 2017. Fort Washington, PA: National Comprehensive Cancer Network. Available at https://www.nccn.org/professionals/physician_gls/pdf/sclc.pdf

Pavel M et al. ENETS consensus guidelines for the management of patients with liver and other distant metastases from neuroendocrine neoplasms of foregut, midgut, hindgut, and unknown primary. Neuroendocrinology. 2012;**95**(2):157–76.

Rekhtman N. Neuroendocrine tumors of the lung: an update. Arch Pathol Lab Med. 2010 Nov;**134**(11):1628–38.

Sayeg Y et al. [Pulmonary neuroendocrine neoplasms]. Pneumologie. 2014 Jul;**68**(7):456–77.

Travis WD, **Brambilla E**, **Burke AP**, **Marx A**, **Nicolson AG**. WHO Classification of Tumours of the Lung, Pleura, Thymus and Heart. Fourth edition. Lyon, France: International Agency for Research on Cancer; 2015.

van Essen M, **Krenning EP**, **Bakker WH**, **de Herder WW**, **van Aken MO**, **Kwekkeboom DJ**. Peptide receptor radionuclide therapy with 177Lu-octreotate in patients with foregut carcinoid tumours of bronchial, gastric and thymic origin. Eur J Nucl Med Mol Imaging. 2007 Aug;**34**(8):1219–27.

Yao JC et al. Everolimus for the treatment of advanced, non-functional neuroendocrine tumours of the lung or gastrointestinal tract (RADIANT-4): a randomised, placebo-controlled, phase 3 study. Lancet. 2016 Mar;**387**(10022):968–77.

Online resources

National Comprehensive Cancer Network

◆ NCCN clinical practice guidelines in oncology: neuroendocrine tumors, https:// www.nccn. org/ professionals/ physician_ gls/ PDF/ neuroendocrine.pdf

UpToDate

◆ Thomas FC et al., Lung neuroendocrine (carcinoid) tumors: Treatment and prognosis, https:// www.uptodate.com/contents/lung-neuroendocrine-carcinoid-tumors-treatment-and-prognosis

◆ Thomas FC et al., Lung neuroendocrine (carcinoid) tumors: Epidemiology, risk factors, classification, histology, diagnosis, and staging, https://www.uptodate.com/contents/lung-neuroendocrine-carcinoid-tumors-epidemiology-risk-factors-classification-histology-diagnosis-and-staging

Case 24

A 54 year old patient with T4N2M0 squamous cell carcinoma who developed neutropenic sepsis during the second course of chemotherapy

Adam Januszewski and Sanjay Popat

Case history

A 54 year old male presented to an accident and emergency department 9 days after commencing his first cycle of second-line chemotherapy for stage IV squamous cell lung cancer. He felt unwell with fever, cough productive of green sputum, and increasing fatigue.

He had been diagnosed with SCC of the right lung invading the mediastinum (T4) with bulky subcarinal lymph nodes (N2). He had undergone six cycles of first-line palliative platinum doublet chemotherapy (gemcitabine–carboplatin) and achieved stable disease for 4 months. He had recently received five fractions of palliative radiotherapy to T8–L2 for difficult to control pain in the context of progressive disease. He had commenced second-line docetaxel (an intravenous taxane chemotherapy) with nintedanib (a multikinase angiogenesis inhibitor). He had COPD, paroxysmal atrial fibrillation, and rheumatoid arthritis.

On attendance at the accident and emergency department he was found to be hypoxic (oxygen saturation 84% on air), febrile (temperature 39.5°C), tachycardic, and hypotensive (heart rate 120/min, blood pressure 90/45 mmHg). He appeared unwell and on auscultation of his chest coarse crepitations were identified at the right lower zone.

Questions

1. What are the first steps in the management of this patient, who is suspected to have neutropenic sepsis?

2. What risk stratification tool can be used to predict the outcome in patients with neutropenic sepsis?

Answers

1. What are the first steps in the management of this patient, who is suspected to have neutropenic sepsis?

The first concern for any doctor who sees a patient on systemic chemotherapy with evidence of infection is neutropenic sepsis. After immediate resuscitation, blood cultures should be drawn before commencing broad spectrum antibiotics (optimally within 1 hour). As in any patient with evidence of infection and systemic compromise, resuscitation, investigation, and antibiotics form the mainstay of treatment. This patient requires cautious oxygen therapy, fluid resuscitation, blood tests (including an urgent full blood count, CRP, and renal and liver blood profile), and blood cultures taken prior to broad spectrum intravenous antibiotics. Antibiotics should not be held waiting for the blood results (specifically the neutrophil count).

2. What risk stratification tool can be used to predict the outcome in patients with neutropenic sepsis?

Fevers in the context of neutropenia can be a life-threatening condition, although in a large proportion of patients febrile neutropenia follows a benign and uncomplicated course. Identifying patients who have a higher chance of complications or death through risk stratification enables better planning for escalation and appropriate levels of care. Patients with thoracic and haematological malignancies have worse outcomes than those with solid organ cancers. However, many patients follow a benign and uncomplicated course and identifying those patients at low risk of complications for an early intravenous to oral antibiotic switch and outpatient management would be beneficial. The above patient would score 12 on the Multinational Association for Supportive Care in Cancer (MASCC) febrile neutropenia risk scoring, which equates to a 36% chance of mortality on this episode.

Neutropenic sepsis

Neutropenia is a well-known and life-threatening side effect for cytotoxic chemotherapies as they inhibit the mitotic ability of the bone marrow and reduce its ability to synthesize haematopoietic cells. Cytotoxic agents prevent the maturation of primitive bone marrow cells and subsequent release of erythrocytes, leucocytes, and platelets. The bone marrow will continue to release mature cells; however, as these pass through their natural life cycle, the blood counts will fall and reach what is known as their 'nadir'. The nadir will depend on the type of cell and treatment regimen, although for neutrophils this is typically between 7 and 10 days after treatment. Differing protocols and agents mean that anyone on systemic treatment should be considered at risk of neutropenia.

Although the laboratory definition of neutropenic sepsis varies, the most common definition is a neutrophil count of <0.5 × 10^9/L and an oral temperature of >38.3°C (or more than two occasions of recording >38°C). Patients who have received vertebral radiotherapy or have bone marrow involvement are at increased risk of developing neutropenia with treatment. Furthermore, patients are at increased risk during their first cycle of the course and if they have had previous exposure to chemotherapy. Other factors that predict neutropenia include tumour type (lung), female sex, advancing age (>65 years), higher performance status, as well as a number of comorbidities.

Recognition and management of neutropenic sepsis

One of the most serious complications of systemic anticancer treatment is neutropenic sepsis. In the National Confidential Enquiry into Patient Outcomes and Death (NCEPOD) report *Systemic Anti-Cancer Therapy: For Better, For Worse?* (Mort et al. 2008) the peak incidence in death after systemic treatment was between 11 and 15 days after chemotherapy and this is likely to be related to neutropenic sepsis. Neutropenia should therefore be suspected in any patient on systemic treatment for cancer. It is typically seen with cytotoxic chemotherapies and occasionally with targeted agents. Although the recognition of infection is the same as in the non-neutropenic patient, sometimes a neutropenic patient can present non-specifically unwell with fatigue as their only complaint. Neutropenic fevers constitute a spectrum of diseases that range from simple and uncomplicated infection through systemic inflammatory response syndrome to severe sepsis—based upon the physiological parameters and organ involvement.

The management of a patient with sepsis is well described and similar to that in the non-neutropenic patient. Management includes aggressive fluid resuscitation and blood tests to assess organ function, full blood count, inflammatory markers, and coagulation. Monitoring of physiological status through urine output, blood pressure, and in some patients central venous pressure monitoring may be required. A source of infection should be sought through a full septic screen to include urinary culture and blood culture (sputum culture) and, should symptoms dictate, further imaging (chest x-ray, abdominal imaging). Specifically in patients with cancer, occasionally there are occult sources of infection as they may have indwelling lines (portacaths, peripherally inserted central catheter lines, Hickman lines), stents (hepatic, renal), as well as the possibility of infection arising from necrotic or fistulating tumours. Currently 70% of pathogens are Gram positive, compared with previously when Gram-negative organisms predominated, and this is likely to be related to indwelling lines and the use of prophylactic antibiotics.

Antibiotic choice should be broad spectrum initially until a source and sensitivities have been identified. Antibiotics administered within an hour of attendance reduce mortality from 60% to 25% (Kumar et al. 2006). Typical antibiotic combinations include broad spectrum penicillin with an aminoglycoside, although local protocols vary according to sensitivities and should be followed. The antibiotic spectrum should subsequently be narrowed if a source/pathogen is identified. In up to 60% of cases a source is never identified (Ahn et al. 2011).

Outcomes and the Multinational Association for Supportive Care in Cancer risk index

Docetaxel in the second-line setting for lung cancer has significant rates of neutropenia (67%), although this translates into only 1.8% of patients with neutropenic sepsis. Patients with lung cancer typically fare less well than those with other tumour sites; this is related to their comorbidities (e.g. chronic obstructive airways disease, ischaemic heart disease) and propensity to pulmonary infection. On multivariate analysis a respiratory rate >24/min, CRP >9.0, platelets <50 000, or a neutropenia lasting ≥4 days were independent predictors of unfavourable outcomes. Furthermore, a MASCC score of <21 was highly significant ($P < 0.001$) for unfavourable outcome despite initially being developed to predict those who will have a favourable outcome. Patients with a neutrophil count <0.1 × 10^9/L have a 20% chance of bacteraemia and a Gram-negative bacteraemia is associated with an 18% mortality (5% in Gram-positive bacteraemia).

The MASCC scoring system was developed to identify low-risk febrile neutropenic patients so that they may be managed in a more convenient or cost-effective way. It is a method of scoring patients based on physiological and biological characteristics assessed on admission and at 24 hours.

Upon initiation of antibiotics international guidelines on the management of patients with sepsis should be adhered to (Surviving Sepsis Campaign); these include lactate measurement and urine output monitoring with catheterization should it be necessary. In patients who fail to respond to resuscitation, escalation to the appropriate level of care may be required to enable central venous pressure monitoring and inotropes to maintain systemic blood pressure and renal perfusion. Escalation of treatment to include antifungals may be appropriate if the patient has had a prolonged duration of neutropenia or there is a high level of clinical suspicion. Gram-negative bacteraemia and MASCC high-risk patients predict for poor outcomes.

Granulocyte–colony stimulating factor: primary and secondary prophylaxis

The use of granulocyte–colony stimulating factor (G-CSF) in patients with febrile neutropenia reduces the duration of neutropenia and hospitalization, although there is insufficient evidence that it improves survival. European Organisation for Research and Treatment of Cancer (EORTC) and ASCO guidelines advise against the routine use of G-CSF as an adjunct to uncomplicated febrile neutropenia. However, it should be considered in patients at high risk of complications (such as those with sepsis or severe sepsis). The use of G-CSF after an episode of febrile neutropenia (secondary prophylaxis) reduces subsequent episodes of febrile neutropenia.

EORTC guidelines advise the use of primary prophylaxis with G-CSF in chemotherapies with a high risk of febrile neutropenia (classified as >20% risk), or those with intermediate risk (10–20%) where patient-related factors may increase the risk of febrile neutropenia (e.g. age, advanced disease, or previous episodes). High-risk chemotherapy schedules in patients with lung cancer include (but the list is not exhaustive) docetaxel–carboplatin, etoposide–cisplatin, and topotecan. G-CSF can also be given to maintain dose intensity. The use of prophylactic G-CSF reduces the relative risk of neutropenia by up to 50%. The use of prophylactic antibiotics (fluoroquinolones) should be restricted to those at high risk of neutropenic sepsis as there is increasing emergence of antibiotic-resistant pathogens that would eventually render any prophylaxis obsolete.

Learning points

◆ Neutropenic sepsis is a well-described, life-threatening complication of chemotherapy in lung cancer and should be considered in all patients with lung cancer on systemic treatment.

◆ Urgent treatment should be instigated that includes resuscitation, broad spectrum antibiotics, and monitoring of physiological variables in the right care setting.

◆ International guidelines for the management of sepsis should be adhered to while being aware that patients who are neutropenic may deteriorate rapidly.

◆ Risk stratification using tools such as MASCC can identify those patients who are at risk of developing a complication of their infection—or those who are at low risk and therefore can be managed with oral antibiotics in the outpatient setting.

◆ Primary prophylaxis with G-CSF and fluoroquinolone antibiotics should be given to all patients with a risk of neutropenic sepsis >20%. Patient and disease risk factors for neutropenia should be considered in other patients receiving regimens with a 10–20% risk of neutropenic sepsis.

References

Ahn S, Lee YS, Chun YH, Kwon IH, Kim W, Lim KS, Kim TW, Lee KH. Predictive factors of poor prognosis in cancer patients with chemotherapy-induced febrile neutropenia. Support Care Cancer. 2011 Aug;**19**(8):1151–8.

Kumar A et al. Duration of hypotension before initiation of effective antimicrobial therapy is the critical determinant of survival in human septic shock. Crit Care Med. 2006 Jun;**34**(6):1589–96.

Mort D, Lansdown M, Smith N, Protopapa K, Mason M. Systemic Anti-Cancer Therapy: For Better, For Worse? London, UK: National Confidential Enquiry into Patient Outcomes and Death; 2008. Available at http://www.ncepod.org.uk/2008sacttoolkit.html

Further reading

Dellinger RP et al. Surviving Sepsis Campaign: international guidelines for management of severe sepsis and septic shock: 2008. Crit Care Med. 2008 Jan;**36**(1):296–327.

Klastersky J et al. The Multinational Association for Supportive Care in Cancer Risk Index: a multinational scoring system for identifying low-risk febrile neutropenic cancer patients. J Clin Oncol. 2000 Aug;**18**(16):3038–51.

Mort D, Lansdown M, Smith N, Protopapa K, Mason M. Systemic Anti-Cancer Therapy: For Better, For Worse? London, UK: National Confidential Enquiry into Patient Outcomes and Death; 2008. Available at http://www.ncepod.org.uk/2008sacttoolkit.html

National Institute for Health and Care Excellence. Neutropenic Sepsis: Prevention and Management in People with Cancer. Clinical Guideline CG151. London, UK: NICE; 2012. Available at https://www.nice.org.uk/guidance/cg151

Case 25

A 76 year old female with an oligometastatic stage IV squamous cell carcinoma who developed diarrhoea on treatment with immune checkpoint inhibitors

Adam Januszewski and Sanjay Popat

Case history

A 76 year old female presented to her GP with a 3 month history of pain in her left leg. She initially noticed pain in her thigh with ambulation, with progressive worsening. She was placed on non-steroidal anti-inflammatory drugs, but there was no improvement. An x-ray of the femur showed a destructive lesion in the diaphysis. A CT scan of the abdomen and chest showed a nodule in the left upper lobe of the lung (Fig. 25.1) and another lesion in segment 6/7 of the liver, suggestive of haemangioma (Fig. 25.2). A bone scan confirmed the lesion in the femur but did not show any other lesions (Fig. 25.3). These findings led to a biopsy of the lesion in the femur. Pathology was consistent with metastatic SCC of the lung.

Questions

1. How will you proceed? Would you request a PET-CT scan of this patient?
2. What is the most appropriate next step?
3. How will you proceed?
4. What is the most appropriate next step?
5. Is a biomarker needed to offer immunotherapy?
6. What treatment does this patient need?
7. How long should you maintain this patient on steroids?
8. Would you consider restarting immunotherapy?

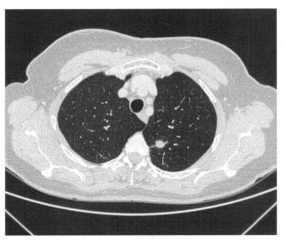

Fig. 25.1 CT chest scan showing a left upper zone nodule.

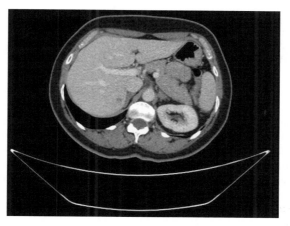

Fig. 25.2 CT scan of the liver showing a lesion suggestive of haemangioma.

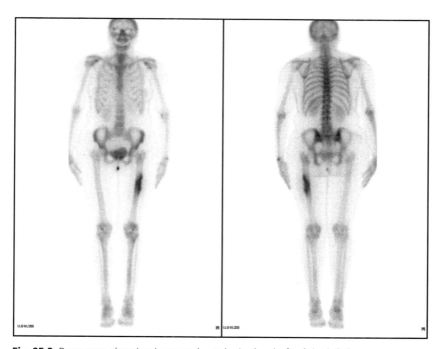

Fig. 25.3 Bone scan showing increased uptake in the shaft of the left femur.

Answers

1. How will you proceed? Would your request a PET-CT scan of this patient?

Oligometastasis occurs in those patients with metastases that are limited in number and location. The number of metastases required to consider the disease as being oligometastatic can vary and has ranged from the presence of a single metastatic lesion to a single organ with multiple metastases or multiple lesions in multiple organs. However, the most commonly accepted number of metastatic lesions considered to constitute an oligometastatic state is up to five, and these should be suitable for radical treatment by local therapy (surgical resection, radiotherapy, or both) to achieve long-term survival. The number of metastatic lesions is an expression of a higher tumour burden and is a potential predictor of survival. Patients with a single lesion have longer survival than those with multiple lesions in one site and those with multiple lesions in multiple sites. Currently, the frequency of a single metastasis in patients with NSCLC is approximately 20–25%.

This subgroup of patients with stage IV NSCLC with a few metastases at diagnosis may be cured with comprehensive radical therapy (surgery or radiotherapy to the primary and the metastases) in addition to systemic treatment. A thorough assessment of the extent of the disease, including PET-CT and brain MRI, should be done to rule out other localizations of metastases.

PET-CT is really important in the decision-making process for a patient with exclusively thoracic disease or oligometastatic disease when radical treatment is indicated. Several studies have shown that PET-CT detects occult metastases in 6–17% of patients with NSCLC that conventional staging methods failed to identify. It is not important to carry out a PET-CT scan in patients with multiple metastases in a single site or in multiple sites detected by CT scan that are not suitable for radical treatment.

Case history continued

A PET-CT scan was performed because the patient had a unique bone lesion. Oligometastatic stage IV disease was suspected and a PET-CT scan was carried out to rule out other metastases. The PET-CT scan confirmed the presence of only the lung lesion and the bone lesion.

2. What is the most appropriate next step?

In patients with oligometastatic disease, treatment with chemotherapy and ablative local therapy such as radiotherapy or surgery to treat the primary lesion and the metastases may enable long-term survival.

Case history continued

The patient suffered a pathological fracture of the femur the day before chemo-therapy was due to commence (Fig. 25.4a). Internal fixation to stabilize the bone lesion was performed (Fig. 25.4b), followed by radical radiotherapy to the bone.

Following radiotherapy to the femur, the patient underwent four cycles of cisplatin–vinorelbine chemotherapy concurrently with thoracic radiotherapy. A chest CT scan carried out at the end of the treatment showed a partial response. The patient's performance status and mobility improved. She did not report any bone pain.

Six months later, the patient presented at the clinic with a 2 week history of right leg oedema. She also complained about asthenia and anorexia.

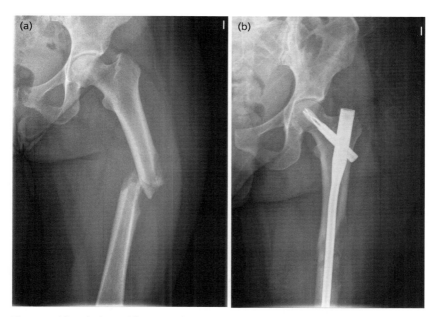

Fig. 25.4 (a) Pathological fracture of the left femur. (b) Internal fixation.

3. How you will proceed?

Patients with cancer may undergo a wasting syndrome characterized by asthenia, anorexia, and loss of weight. The presence of these symptoms makes it necessary to rule out disease progression. In addition, in this patient with leg oedema, deep vein thrombosis should also be ruled out. Patients with cancer are at risk of thrombotic complications due to a hypercoagulable state. Clinical venous thromboembolism (VTE) occurs in approximately 10% of patients with cancer. The risk factors for VTE are: tumour-specific factors (procoagulant activity induced by the tumour cells and non-cancerous tissues); anatomical factors (compression or invasion of vessels, etc.); patient-specific factors (obesity, advanced age, etc.); and factors associated with the treatment (chemotherapy, high-risk surgery, etc.).

A body CT scan and a leg US are indicated in this patient.

Case history continued

The US was normal; there was no thrombosis on the images. However, the CT scan showed disease progression: lung left hilar consolidation (Fig. 25.5a); mediastinal, left axillar (31 mm), retroperitoneal (10.5–13.4 mm), and left iliac (11.5–16.6 mm) lymph node enlargement; and a right suprarenal mass (51.8 mm). Lymphoedema secondary to iliac burden disease was diagnosed.

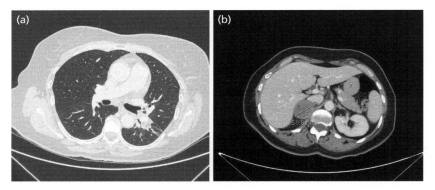

Fig. 25.5 (a) CT chest scan showing a left hilar mass. (b) CT scan of the abdomen showing a large right adrenal mass.

4. What is the most appropriate next step?

The patient has a stage IV lung cancer with multiple metastases progressing at 6 months after the end of first-line chemotherapy. No curative options exist in this setting. Second-line therapy for patients with NSCLC with a squamous histology has been docetaxel or erlotinib. However, recently, the FDA withdrew the indication of erlotinib in patients with wild-type EGFR. Immune checkpoint inhibitors such as anti-PD-1 inhibitors (nivolumab and pembrolizumab) or anti-PD-L1 inhibitor (atezolizumab) were superior to docetaxel in a second-line setting in adenocarcinoma or squamous cell lung cancer. Other immunotherapeutic agents, as well as combinations of some of these or with chemotherapy, are being tested.

Case history continued

The patient was offered the opportunity to participate in a clinical trial comparing chemotherapy with immunotherapy. The patient was randomized and allocated to the tremelimumab (anti-CTLA-4 antibody) and durvalumab (anti-PD-L1 antibody) arm of the trial.

5. Is a biomarker needed to offer immunotherapy?

The use of biomarkers for immunotherapy remains controversial. PD-L1 expression by IHC is the most commonly used biomarker because increasing tumour PD-L1 expression has been correlated with benefit from anti-PD-1 or anti-PD-L1 treatment. However, several antibodies and different thresholds of positivity have been used in clinical trials. Moreover, heterogeneity is a common characteristic of tumours and different expressions of PD-L1 have been seen in different areas of tumours as well as at different times in the evolution of a disease.

Case history continued

PD-L1 IHC was negative in this patient. She started treatment with a combination of tremelimumab and durvalumab. Following two cycles of treatment there was a reduction in the lung infiltrate (Fig. 25.6a), the mediastinal nodes disappeared, and the adrenal mass (Fig. 25.6b) and iliac nodes (partial response) were reduced in size. The patient showed really good tolerance. However, after the third cycle of treatment she developed a fever and grade 3 diarrhoea and was admitted to hospital.

6. What treatment does this patient need?

Immunotherapy is associated with a different safety profile from chemotherapy. The specific effects are immune-related adverse events (irAEs), which reflect the immune-based mechanism of action of checkpoint inhibitors. The most common irAEs are skin and gastrointestinal tract toxicity, although the liver, endocrine system, and other organs may also be affected. The rates of high-grade irAEs (grade 3–4) are higher for anti-PD-1 antibodies combined with anti-CTLA-4 treatment than for anti-PD-L-1 or anti-CTLA-4 monotherapy.

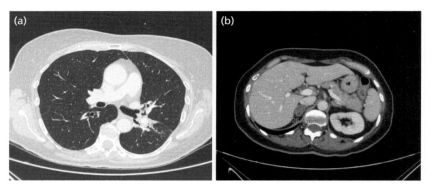

Fig. 25.6 (a) CT chest scan showing a reduction in the left hilar mass. (b) CT scan of the abdomen showing a reduction in the right adrenal mass.

Gastrointestinal tract toxicity is commonly reported with immunotherapy, and includes diarrhoea, colitis, and enteritis. According to the National Cancer Institute's common terminology criteria for adverse events, colitis refers to abdominal pain, bloody stools, or peritoneal signs, whereas diarrhoea is based on stool frequency alone. Enteritis is associated with symptoms similar to colitis, but the inflammation involves the small bowel. Classification of the severity of diarrhoea and its appropriate management is as follows:

◆ Grade 1: <4 stools per day over baseline. A complete blood test and stool laboratory tests should be carried out to rule out other causes (*Clostridium difficile*, parasites, etc.). Immunotherapy can be continued and corticosteroids are not indicated.

◆ Grade 2: 4–6 stools per day over baseline with blood or mucus in the stool. The same laboratory tests are needed as for grade 1. Immunotherapy must be stopped until there is resolution to grade 0–1. Colonoscopy and biopsy should be considered if the diagnosis is unclear. Patients should be monitored and encouraged to report worsening symptoms immediately. Systemic corticosteroids should also be considered.

◆ Grade 3 or 4: >7 stools per day over baseline, fever, and peritoneal signs. The same laboratory tests are needed as for grade 1. Immunotherapy must be stopped until there is resolution to grade 0–1. Systemic corticosteroids are required. If patients do not respond to steroids, infliximab must be considered.

Case history continued

A stool study, abdominal x-ray, and complete blood test were performed. Intravenous hydration, antibiotics, and systemic steroids were initiated. When the patient was clinically stable a sigmoidoscopy was performed.

7. How long should you maintain this patient on steroids?

Waxing and waning of symptoms is common, and severe courses of systemic corticosteroids over no less than 30 days may be required. Steroids should be continued until grade 1 or 0 toxicity is reached, followed by a taper over at least 30 days.

If symptoms do not improve with steroids after 72 hours of treatment, the tumour necrosis factor-α blocking agent infliximab (5 mg/kg once every 2 weeks) may be used, but not in patients with gastrointestinal perforation or sepsis. Infliximab usually improves gastrointestinal adverse events within 24 hours.

Case history continued

The patient improved with systemic corticosteroids within 72 hours. After 15 days oral steroids were started and tapered over the next 15 days. The patient was discharged from the hospital.

8. Would you considered restarting immunotherapy?

Most protocols recommend discontinuing immunotherapy with this level of diarrhoea.

Further reading

Hellwig D, Ukena D, Paulsen F, Bamberg M, Kirsch CM; Onko-PET der Deutschen Gesellschaft fur Nuklearmedizin. Meta-analysis of the efficacy of positron emission tomography with F-18-fluorodeoxyglucose in lung tumors. Basis for discussion of the German Consensus Conference on PET in Oncology 2000. Pneumologie. 2001 Aug;**55**(8):367–77.

Ouyang WW, Su SF, Ma Z, Hu YX, Lu B, Li QS, Geng YC, Li HQ. Prognosis of non-small cell lung cancer patients with bone oligometastases treated concurrently with thoracic three-dimensional radiotherapy and chemotherapy. Radiat Oncol. 2014 Jun;**9**:147.

Villadolid J, Amin A. Immune checkpoint inhibitors in clinical practice: update on management of immune-related toxicities. Transl Lung Cancer Res. 2015 Oct;**4**(5):560–75.

Weber JS, Kähler KC, Hauschild A. Management of immune-related adverse events and kinetics of response with ipilimumab. J Clin Oncol. 2012 Jul;**30**(21):2691–7.

Weber JS, Postow M, Lao CD, Schadendorf D. Management of adverse events following treatment with anti-programmed death-1 agents. Oncologist. 2016 Oct;**21**(10):1230–40.

Case 26

A 55 year old female with relapsed stage IV ALK fusion-positive adenocarcinoma treated with crizotinib, presenting with headaches

Adam Januszewski and Sanjay Popat

Case history

A 55 year old female with no history of smoking presented as an emergency with shortness of breath over the previous 2 weeks. During the hours before her arrival at the accident and emergency department, she experienced increased shortness of breath and the onset of pleuritic pain. Physical examination revealed a blood pressure of 100/70 mmHg, heart rate of 85/min, and a respiratory rate of 24/min. The patient was pale and diaphoretic. Chest x-rays showed an enlarged cardiac shape and an electrocardiogram showed ST elevation and low QRS voltage in the precordial leads. An echocardiogram showed a large pericardial effusion with cardiac tamponade physiology. She was referred to the intensive care unit and a pericardial drainage tube was placed.

The pericardial fluid sent for cytology confirmed adenocarcinoma. A chest, abdomen, and pelvis CT scan showed bilateral pulmonary nodules and liver metastases. On the basis of these findings the patient was diagnosed with lung adenocarcinoma stage IV (pulmonary and hepatic metastases). Molecular testing revealed the presence of an ALK rearrangement but no EGFR mutation.

Questions

1. Would you recommend a PET-CT scan for this patient?
2. What is known about serous involvement in ALK-positive NSCLC?
3. What is the most appropriate next step?
4. What is the suspected diagnosis?
5. What examination would you request for this patient?
6. What is the most appropriate next step?
7. What would you recommend for this patient?

Answers

1. Would you recommend a PET/CT scan for this patient?

PET-CT is emerging as a potential diagnosis and staging test in patients with lung cancer. It combines anatomical information from a CT scan with metabolic information from PET. PET-CT offers the highest sensitivity for mediastinal lymph nodes and distant metastasis assessment, except for the brain.

When metastatic disease appears on a CT scan of the chest and upper abdomen or on brain imaging, other imaging is only necessary when it might impact treatment such as in patients with oligometastatic disease who could be managed with radical treatment. Current NICE guidelines do not recommend PET-CT imaging in the palliative (non-radical) setting.

2. What is known about serous involvement in ALK-positive NSCLC?

Pericardial effusion is commonly associated with malignancy; lung and breast cancer are the most common causes of malignant pericardial effusions. NSCLC with ALK gene rearrangements is significantly associated with pericardial and pleural involvement and effusions.

3. What is the most appropriate next step?

ALK rearrangements are reported in about 3–7% of NSCLCs. Determination of the EGFR and ALK status is recommended in patients with NSCLC and an adenocarcinoma histology. Crizotinib has shown better efficacy and tolerability in patients with NSCLC and ALK rearrangement than chemotherapy.

In a phase III trial in patients previously treated with chemotherapy who then relapsed, crizotinib compared with second-line chemotherapy showed a significantly increased progression-free survival (median 7.7 versus 3 months) and response rate (60% versus 20%). No significant difference in overall survival was observed (median 20.3 versus 22.8 months), primarily because 64% of chemotherapy-treated patients received crizotinib after progressing.

A second trial (PROFILE 1014) compared crizotinib with standard platinum-based doublet chemotherapy as the first-line treatment in patients with advanced ALK-positive NSCLC. Patients randomized to the chemotherapy group were allowed to cross over to crizotinib upon progression. The study achieved its primary endpoint, with a significant improvement in progression-free survival in the crizotinib arm (median 10.9 versus 7 months). The median overall survival for both arms was not reached, but was markedly better than historical rates for chemotherapy.

On the basis of the results of these trials crizotinib is preferred as the initial therapy for patients with tumours containing an ALK rearrangement.

Case history continued

Owing to the patient's condition, she began treatment with platinum-based doublet chemotherapy (carboplatin–paclitaxel) before the results of the ALK test were available. Her performance status improved, but unfortunately disease progression was detected after three cycles.

She started treatment with crizotinib with a good response and good tolerability. After 1 year of treatment she presented with headaches over the course of 2 weeks.

4. What is the suspected diagnosis?

Despite the good initial response, the majority of patients with lung cancer and ALK rearrangements treated with crizotinib will relapse within 12 months owing to the development of secondary resistance. Moreover, the efficacy of crizotinib has not translated to the control of intracranial disease. The CNS is frequently a site of disease progression: up to 60% of patients develop metastases during treatment with crizotinib. In the case of CNS disease, progression is attributable to both poor intracranial penetration of the drugs and the emergence of intrinsic tumour resistance mechanisms.

In this patient the appearance of headaches after 1 year of treatment is suspicious for the development of brain metastases. Other possibilities such as infections and secondary effects of treatment should be excluded.

5. What examination would you request for this patient?

MRI has an established role for distinguishing malignant lesions from benign lesions and it is more accurate than brain CT for the diagnosis of brain metastases. Contrast-enhanced brain CT can be carried out as a valid alternative if there are contraindications to MRI or it is not available.

Case history continued

MRI showed multiple brain metastases (Fig. 26.1).

6. What is the most appropriate next step?

Relapse with brain metastases is a particular problem in patients with stage IV NSCLC and ALK rearrangements treated with crizotinib. There may be different clinical scenarios with different treatment approaches, including the following.

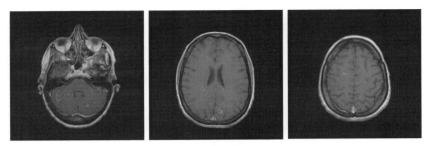

Fig. 26.1 MRI of the head showing brain metastasis.

- Brain oligoprogression. Extracranial disease is controlled and there is isolated brain progression. In this setting, continuation of treatment with crizotinib after treatment for the brain metastases with radiotherapy or surgery is recommended and may be associated with a significant interval free of progression of the extracranial disease.
- Systemic and brain progression. Treatment of the brain metastases and switching to a second-generation ALK inhibitor is recommended.

Ceritinib and alectinib are second-generation ALK inhibitors that have activity in crizotinib-resistant disease. Ceritinib showed a response rate of 56% in patients previously treated with crizotinib and 72% in ALK inhibitor-naive patients. Ceritinib has demonstrated response rates of 50% in patients with crizotinib-resistant disease.

In addition, other ALK inhibitors such as brigatinib and lorlatinib have shown promising activity in crizotinib-refractory disease. Differential sensitivity has been observed between these ALK inhibitors, depending on the type of ALK mutation associated with resistance to previous ALK inhibitor therapy. Moreover, ceritinib, alectinib, brigatinib, and lorlatinib have all been reported to have activity against brain metastases, including in those patients treated with chemotherapy and crizotinib.

Case history continued

A CT scan was performed, which did not show any extracranial progression.

7. What would you recommend for this patient?

TKIs have improved the outcome in patients with ALK rearrangements; however, treatment of brain metastases remains a challenge. Brain metastases are the usual place of disease progression in patients treated with the first-generation TKI crizotinib.

The majority of patients with brain metastases are treated with whole brain radiation therapy (WBRT). Nowadays, patients could also be treated with radiosurgery alone or in combination with WBRT. Radiotherapy remains an important technique for local control of disease. The combination has shown increased control of brain metastases. On the one hand, because there are limited numbers of brain metastases that are suitable for treatment with radiosurgery, it has little impact on overall survival. On the other hand, WBRT alone, without radiosurgery or surgery, has suboptimal local control and should be used when there are a large number of metastases.

The second-generation ALK inhibitors ceritinib and alectinib have shown good penetration in the CNS. However, the optimal sequence of TKI and brain radiation has yet to be determined. Some authors claim that there is a synergistic effect between radiotherapy and TKIs on local control and the prevention of extracranial disease progression. Nevertheless toxicity may increase.

Follow-up and outcome

Because of the large number of brain metastases WBRT was administrated. The patient was also included in a clinical trial with alectinib 600 mg twice a day. A partial systemic and brain response was attained with excellent tolerance to treatment (Fig. 26.2).

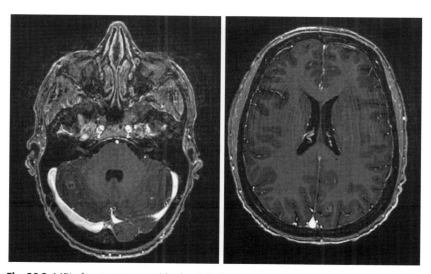

Fig. 26.2 MRI after treatment with alectinib demonstrating a good intracranial response.

Further reading

Aoyama H et al. Stereotactic radiosurgery plus whole-brain radiation therapy vs stereotactic radiosurgery alone for treatment of brain metastases: a randomized controlled trial. JAMA. 2006 Jun;**295**(21):2483–91.

Chuang JC, Neal JW. Crizotinib as first line therapy for advanced *ALK*-positive non-small cell lung cancers. Transl Lung Cancer Res. 2015 Oct;**4**(5):639–41.

Gainor JF, Sherman CA, Willoughby K, Logan J, Kennedy E, Brastianos PK, Chi AS, Shaw AT. Alectinib salvages CNS relapses in ALK-positive lung cancer patients previously treated with crizotinib and ceritinib. J Thorac Oncol. 2015 Feb;**10**(2):232–6.

Solomon BJ et al. First-line crizotinib versus chemotherapy in ALK-positive lung cancer. N Engl J Med. 2014 Dec;**371**:2167–77.

Takeda M, Okamoto I, Nakagawa K. Clinical impact of continued crizotinib administration after isolated central nervous system progression in patients with lung cancer positive for ALK rearrangement. J Thorac Oncol. 2013 May;**8**(5):654–7.

Section III

Clinical oncology

Case 27

Drop metastasis

Andrew Ho and Julian Singer

Case history

A 64 year old female ex-smoker presented 4 years previously with a dry cough and haemoptysis. She had a past medical history of hypertension, hypercholester-olaemia, asthma, and stable chronic kidney disease stage 3. She was treated for a left upper lobe T2N2M0 adenocarcinoma with radical radiotherapy of 55 Gy in 20 once daily fractions over 4 weeks.

Two years later she developed headaches, nausea, and visual disturbance. MRI of the brain was performed (Fig. 27.1).

Questions

1. What does the MRI scan show?
2. What are the treatment options?
3. What would the next step in her management be?
4. What does the MRI scan of the patient's spine show? What is the differential diagnosis? What neurological signs and symptoms might you expect?
5. What are the next steps in this patient's management?
6. What would you do now?

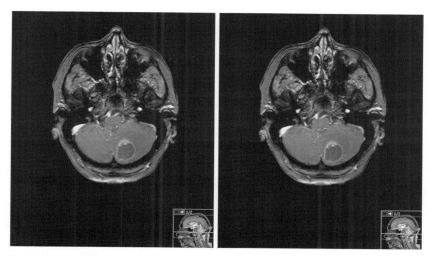

Fig. 27.1 MRI of the head in a patient with headaches, nausea, and visual disturbances and a history of lung cancer.

Answers

1. What does the MRI scan show?

Gadolinium-enhanced T1 (left) and T2 fluid-attenuated inversion recovery (FLAIR) (right) images show a left cerebellar hemisphere ring-enhancing cystic lesion with an enhancing solid component anteriorly. There is surrounding vasogenic oedema. There is a resultant mass effect with partial effacement of the fourth ventricle. The appearances are consistent with a solitary metastasis in the left cerebellar hemisphere.

2. What are the treatment options?

In the first instance, the patient should be started on high-dose steroids (with proton pump inhibitor (PPI) cover and blood glucose monitoring) to reduce peritumoral oedema. There are four main treatment options, which will be discussed in turn: neurosurgical resection; stereotactic radiosurgery; whole brain radiotherapy; and supportive care alone.

1. *Neurosurgical resection.* In patients with a good performance status, controlled extracranial disease, and intracranial disease for which surgical resection is technically feasible, a neurosurgical opinion should be obtained. Clearly, surgery carries a risk of significant peri- and postoperative morbidity and mortality. Therefore, patients should be carefully selected and appropriately counselled.

2. *Stereotactic radiosurgery.* This involves the use of hypofractionated radiotherapy with a high degree of geometric accuracy to deliver an ablative dose. In the UK, there are two platforms commonly used for this. The Elekta Gamma Knife uses a circular array of 201 ^{60}Co sources in a shielded assembly. The patient wears a special frame fixed to the skull, which ensures geometric precision; a single fraction of radiotherapy at an ablative dose is delivered to the tumour. Alternatively, the CyberKnife system uses a 6 MV linear accelerator mounted on a robotic arm with built-in image guidance, negating the need for a surgical frame.

3. *Whole brain radiotherapy (WBRT).* This is perhaps the most widely used treatment carried out by clinical oncologists in this scenario. It can provide rapid improvement in symptoms and allow steroids to be weaned, particularly in patients in whom neurosurgery or stereotactic radiosurgery are not appropriate. Because of the acute toxicity of WBRT, patient selection remains important. The Radiation Therapy Oncology Group recursive partitioning analysis (RPA) (Gaspar et al. 1997) divides patients into prognostic categories and has been used to select those patients who might benefit most from WBRT, although response to steroids and performance status are also considered important factors. WBRT is delivered using opposing lateral fields. A CT planning scan of the head is used to virtually set up the field arrangement. Anatomically, the Reid baseline is used

as the inferior border of the field (supraorbital ridge to external auditory meatus), with care taken to shield the lens. The dose prescription is commonly 20 Gy/5 fractions/1 week, although 30 Gy in 10 fractions is a suitable alternative dose for patients of good performance status.

Recently, there has been some debate on the benefit of WBRT in patients with metastatic non-small-cell lung cancer (NSCLC). The Medical Research Council's QUARTZ trial was a non-inferiority trial randomizing patients with cerebral metastases from NSCLC to supportive care or supportive care plus WBRT (20 Gy/5 fractions/1 week) (Mulvenna et al. 2016). This showed no difference in overall survival, overall quality of life, or dexamethasone usage between the groups. However, it has been suggested that selecting patients with good performance status and RPA class 1 may reveal a difference, and therefore extrapolating the QUARTZ data to different patient groups should be done with caution (only 6% of patients in the trial were RPA class 1).

4. *Supportive management.* Regardless of which of the above three modalities is used, the patient must inform the Driver & Vehicle Licensing Agency and stop driving. Steroids should be weaned as tolerated to avoid the toxicity of prolonged high doses. Prophylactic antiepileptic drugs (AEDs) are unlikely to be of benefit (Mikkelsen et al. 2010), but can be started if the patient has seizures. None of the AEDs have been shown to be more effective than the others, and so levetiracetam, which has minimal drug interactions and a favourable toxicity profile, is a popular choice.

Case history continued

The patient proceeded to have neurosurgical resection of the left cerebellar metastasis.

3. What would the next step in her management be?

There is level I evidence in favour of WBRT following surgical resection (compared with surgical resection alone) (Kalkanis et al. 2010). This reduces local recurrence, as well as recurrence anywhere else in the brain.

However, the combination approach can increase toxicity. If margins are clear a watch and wait approach can be adopted.

Case history continued

Two years later the patient reported weight loss and back pain. An MRI scan of her spine was performed (Fig. 27.2).

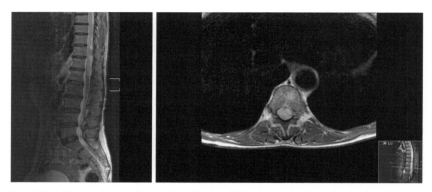

Fig. 27.2 MRI scan in a patient with a history of lung cancer presenting with weight loss and back pain.

4. What does the MRI scan of the patient's spine show? What is the differential diagnosis? What neurological signs and symptoms might you expect?

T2 sagittal and axial images show an intradural extramedullary soft tissue mass compressing the posterior aspect of the dorsal spinal cord at T11. Ordinarily, this would be in keeping with a meningioma. However, given the history of NSCLC with previous surgery to the posterior fossa, drop metastasis is also in the differential. Drop metastases are well-documented but rare sequelae of cerebral metastases with spread via cerebrospinal fluid; neurosurgical intervention is thought to increase the likelihood of drop metastases.

Metastatic spinal cord compression is an oncological emergency. It is usually caused by a crush fracture with or without soft tissue tumour extension, but occasionally it can be a direct extension of malignant lymphadenopathy or an extradural tumour mass causing cord compression without bone involvement. Early stage compression of the spinal cord results in oedema, venous congestion, and demyelination; continued compression causes secondary vascular injury and irreversible infarction. Symptoms and signs will depend on the level of cord compression, but it should be noted that the dermatomal sensory level may be out by several levels from the anatomical compression level. Pain is the most frequent first symptom and often precedes the diagnosis by 3–5 months. Motor weakness often occurs before sensory loss. Autonomic dysfunction is a late complication. Cord compression can also be asymptomatic.

Note that this MRI scan is not typical for classical metastatic spinal cord compression which, as stated above, more often compresses the cord anteriorly. In this case, one might expect the first clinical sign to be damage to the dorsal column–medial lemniscus pathway with resultant loss of fine touch and proprioception. Motor weakness with upper motor neuron signs resulting from compression of the corticospinal tract may well be a later sign, with relative preservation of the spinothalamic tract.

5. What are the next steps in this patient's management?

The patient should be started on high-dose steroids (e.g. dexamethasone 16 mg/day) with PPI cover, blood sugar monitoring, and prophylactic low molecular weight heparin to reduce the risk of thromboembolic disease if not contraindicated. A restaging CT scan should be carried out as this will inform prognosis and therefore suitability for surgical intervention. The best outcomes are with surgical decompression followed by radiotherapy, and the patient should therefore be discussed with a local neurosurgical unit. In this case, it would also be helpful to obtain tissue for histological analysis of the intradural extramedullary lesion.

Surgery in metastatic spinal cord compression should be particularly considered:

◆ if there is a single site of cord compression
◆ if cord compression progresses during radiotherapy or there is recurrence after radiotherapy
◆ if there are radioresistant tumours
◆ if there is a fracture dislocation or an unstable spine
◆ to provide tissue if necessary from a diagnostic perspective (e.g. cancer of an unknown primary where metastatic spinal cord compression is the initial presentation).

Case history continued

The patient proceeded to have a thoracic laminectomy and excision of the T11 tumour. Intraoperatively, the tumour was found to be adherent to the spinal cord with engorged vessels; 95% of the tumour was resected, but a small adherent part was left on the cord.

6. What would you do now?

The patient should receive postoperative radiotherapy as soon as practically possible. Typical prescription is 20 Gy/5 fractions/1 week, prescribed to an appropriate depth as measured on the planning CT (e.g. 7 cm) (Fig. 27.3). The superior and inferior limits of the field are the intervertebral disc encompassing one vertebra superior to and one inferior to the level of compression; this practice reflects the days before availability of CT simulation to ensure that the level of compression was well covered as well as the need for a margin surrounding the target and avoiding the field edge going through a vertebral body. The centre of the field is in the midline along the spinous processes with the width of the transverse processes included (usually 8 cm width). A single posterior field of 6 MV photons is used, with notice taken of the exit beam passing through the liver and gastric regions, which may contribute to acute toxicity of nausea and vomiting.

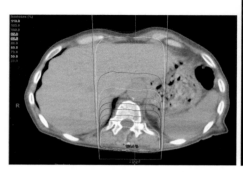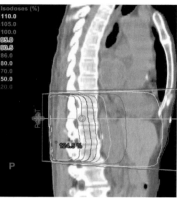

Fig. 27.3 CT planning for thoracic spine radiotherapy.

References

Gaspar L, Scott C, Rotman M, Asbell S, Phillips T, Wasserman T, McKenna WG, Byhardt R. Recursive partitioning analysis (RPA) of prognostic factors in three Radiation Therapy Oncology Group (RTOG) brain metastases trials. Int J Radiat Oncol Biol Phys. 1997 Mar;**37**(4):745–51.

Kalkanis SN et al. The role of surgical resection in the management of newly diagnosed brain metastases: a systematic review and evidence-based clinical practice guideline. J Neurooncol. 2010 Jan;**96**(1):33–43.

Mikkelsen T et al. The role of prophylactic anticonvulsants in the management of brain metastases: a systematic review and evidence-based clinical practice guideline. J Neurooncol. 2010 Jan;**96**(1):97–102.

Mulvenna P et al. Dexamethasone and supportive care with or without whole brain radiotherapy in treating patients with non-small cell lung cancer with brain metastases unsuitable for resection or stereotactic radiotherapy (QUARTZ): results from a phase 3, non-inferiority, randomised trial. Lancet. 2016 Oct;**388**(10055):2004–14.

Case 28

Superior vena cava obstruction due to lung cancer

Andrew Ho and Julian Singer

Case history

A 74 year old female presented to an accident and emergency department with a 2 week history of facial and neck swelling and distended neck veins; this was on the background of a 4 month history of cough, anorexia, and weight loss. She had stopped smoking 6 weeks prior to presentation. A CT scan of the thorax with contrast was performed (Fig. 28.1).

Questions

1. What does the CT scan show?
2. What is the likely diagnosis?
3. What are the presenting symptoms and clinical signs associated with this condition?
4. How would you manage this patient?
5. What are the different treatment options?
6. You decide to give the patient radiotherapy. How would you deliver this, and what side effects may the patient expect?

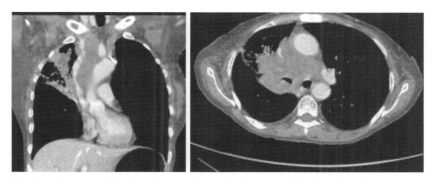

Fig. 28.1 CT scan of the chest in a patient with a history of facial and neck swelling.

Answers

1. What does the CT scan show?

There is a large low-density paramediastinal mass in the right upper lobe extending into the mediastinum with adjacent consolidative changes. There is resultant severe narrowing of the superior vena cava, as well as narrowing of the right pulmonary artery and right main bronchus.

2. What is the likely diagnosis?

The most likely diagnosis is a primary lung cancer causing superior vena cava obstruction (SVCO), probably of small-cell or squamous cell histology. Other malignant causes of SVCO include lymphoma (more common with non-Hodgkin lymphoma than with Hodgkin lymphoma); rarely, these are thymoma and germ cell tumours.

3. What are the presenting symptoms and clinical signs associated with this condition?

The onset of SVCO symptoms is typically insidious over weeks, but it can present with sudden occlusion or with associated airway obstruction. Patients can report dyspnoea, cough, neck/facial swelling, dilated veins overlying the chest wall, headache, nasal congestion, epistaxis, dizziness, and syncope. Bending forwards can exacerbate symptoms. They may also have symptoms representative of their primary malignancy and/or metastatic disease (e.g. haemoptysis, anorexia, weight loss).

Clinical examination shows fixed raised external jugular veins bilaterally, venous collaterals in the distribution of the superior vena cava, facial swelling, bilateral arm oedema, plethora, and papilloedema (a late sign). The Pemberton manoeuvre involves elevating both arms until they touch the sides of the head. This results in facial plethora due to obstruction of the thoracic inlet.

4. How would you manage this patient?

Immediate management involves sitting the patient up and providing supplementary oxygen if required. The patient should be started on high-dose steroids (dexamethasone 8 mg twice daily) with PPI cover and blood glucose monitoring. If the patient is severely compromised then consider concomitant tracheal compression. Investigations include chest x-ray (showing a widened mediastinum) followed by a CT scan with contrast to demonstrate the site and cause of SVCO; the CT scan will also act as the baseline staging and imaging for post-treatment comparison. This can also show an intraluminal thrombus, which should be treated with anticoagulation if present. If the patient's clinical condition allows the time for it, a histological diagnosis should be sought prior to definitive treatment (e.g. by endobronchial ultrasound or CT-guided biopsy).

5. What are the different treatment options?

There have historically been three treatment modalities used (either alone or in combination) for SVCO: chemotherapy, radiotherapy, and stents. Factors affecting a decision between modalities include tumour histology, stage, performance status, severity of symptoms, and service availability. Chemotherapy has traditionally been considered for tumour types that are particularly chemosensitive (such as small-cell lung cancer (SCLC), germ cell tumours, and lymphoma); symptomatic response rates are of the order of objective response rates. Radiotherapy, when used for SVCO in lung cancer, can provide similar symptomatic response rates to chemotherapy. High-dose steroids are often used in conjunction with radiotherapy because of concerns regarding peritumoral oedema exacerbating the degree of obstruction at the start of treatment. Stent insertion prior to radiotherapy is preferred as it provides a more rapid relief in a high proportion of patients. However, sometimes it is limited by the availability of interventional radiology services. If necessary, following venography thrombolysis can be performed.

6. You decide to give the patient radiotherapy. How would you deliver this, and what side effects would you counsel the patient regarding?

If patients can tolerate it, they are simulated and treated in the supine position with their arms by their sides (alternatively, a sitting position can be used with a single anterior field). Treatment is delivered with parallel opposed anterior and posterior fields. Using a planning CT with virtual simulation, the field should encompass the tumour, mediastinum, and superior vena cava; a field size of approximately 12 × 12 cm is typical (Fig. 28.2). Palliative regimens include 20 Gy/5 fractions/1 week or 30 Gy/10 fractions/2 weeks. In patients with a poor performance status and prognosis, symptomatic relief can be provided with more hypofractionated regimens (e.g. 10 Gy/1 fraction or 16 Gy/2 fractions), although there is a risk of increasing oedema.

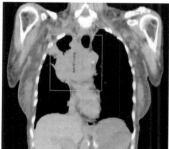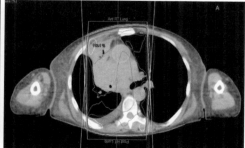

Fig. 28.2 CT planning scan for radiotherapy.

Depending on the dose fractionation used, patients can experience fatigue, skin soreness, local hair loss, respiratory symptoms (shortness of breath, infection), and sore swallowing. Steroids are used to minimize any temporary worsening of symptoms but patients should be warned regarding this. They should also be aware that a lack of symptomatic relief and relapse are both possible.

Case history continued

Following radiotherapy, the patient's scan showed a good response in the lungs (Fig. 28.3). A CT-guided biopsy showed SCLC. However, the patient had progression with pleural effusion and liver metastases.

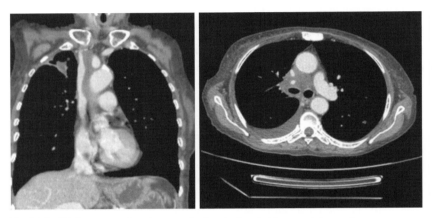

Fig. 28.3 CT chest scan showing a reduction in the right upper lobe and mediastinal mass.

7. What would you do next?

The patient should be assessed for fitness for systemic treatment. First-line treatment should be commenced as soon as medically possible. Chemotherapy drugs that are used would be either cisplatin or carboplatin in combination with etoposide. (For further discussion on this topic, see Section II.)

Further reading

Rowell NP, Gleeson FV. Steroids, radiotherapy, chemotherapy and stents for superior vena caval obstruction in carcinoma of the bronchus. Clin Oncol (R Coll Radiol). 2002 Oct;**14**(5):338–51.

Case 29

Pancoast tumour

Kobika Sritharan and Julian Singer

Case history

A 66 year old female ex-smoker presented to her GP with a 3 month history of pain in her left shoulder radiating to her left scapula and down her left arm. She denied any symptoms of cough, haemoptysis, shortness of breath, or weight loss. She had an Eastern Cooperative Oncology Group (ECOG) performance status of 0. Her GP referred her to the respiratory rapid access clinic and the following images were taken (Fig. 29.1).

Questions

1. What syndrome may be present and what signs should the physician look for in this patient?

2. Which American radiologist first described this type of tumour?

3. What further investigations should be organized to establish diagnosis and stage?

4. Is there local extension of this tumour?

5. How would you manage this patient and what are her treatment options?

6. What are the further management options for this patient?

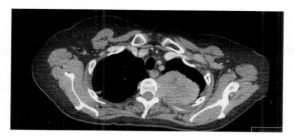

Fig. 29.1 CT scan of the chest showing a left upper lobe mass.

Answers

1. What syndrome may be present and what signs should the physician look for in this patient?

Horner syndrome may be present; signs: ipsilateral miosis (constricted pupil), partial ptosis of the eyelid, anhidrosis (reduced sweating on skin of ipsilateral face), and apparent enophthalmos.

2. Which American radiologist first described this type of tumour?

The term Pancoast tumour is attributed to Henry Pancoast, professor of radiology in Pennsylvania, who is thought to have first described this lung cancer in 1932.

3. What further investigations should be organized to establish diagnosis and stage?

Tissue diagnosis is required and the method should be discussed at the multidisciplinary team (MDT) meeting. Biopsy is likely to be by either bronchoscopy or CT-directed biopsy depending on the location of the tumour.

Case history continued

CT-guided biopsy revealed a poorly differentiated adenocarcinoma that was EGFR and anaplastic lymphoma kinase (ALK) mutation negative. A PET scan was performed (Fig. 29.2) to establish whether the patient was suitable for radiotherapy with radical intent or surgery.

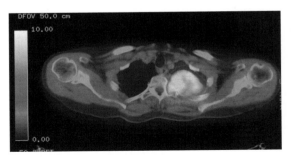

Fig. 29.2 PET-CT scan for staging of lung cancer.

4. Is there local extension of this tumour?

The tumour is extending to and involving the body of the vertebra and the first left rib. This makes it T4 disease. Furthermore a PET scan revealed that her left hilar node was avid therefore she was staged as T4N1M0.

5. How would you manage this patient and what are her treatment options?

The patient's symptoms should be immediately palliated. Often opiates and nerve-modulating analgesics or corticosteroids are effective. She may be treated with palliative radiotherapy. Higher radiation doses are often required for good palliation of pain. She may be suitable for a combination of chemotherapy and radiotherapy with radical intent, or a combination of chemoradiation to down-stage this disease followed by surgical excision in some circumstances. Surgical excision may be possible with removal of the tumour and adjacent rib. Vertebral surgery is possible in some conditions. The patient's overall fitness as well as her wishes should be taken into account when deciding between the treatment options.

Case history continued

The patient was initially treated with two cycles of cisplatin and pemetrexed chemotherapy to cytoreduce the tumour volume in order to facilitate the use of radical radiotherapy. Her pain levels drastically reduced in this time and her performance status improved to 0.

A new CT scan of the thorax (Fig. 29.3) was performed to assess and enable planning for radical radiotherapy. This demonstrated a good partial response.

The patient underwent a 4 week course of radical radiotherapy, with care taken to avoid the organs at risk such as the spinal cord, followed by two further cycles of chemotherapy. A new CT scan (Fig. 29.4) showed a further partial response of the tumour and no apparent lymphadenopathy.

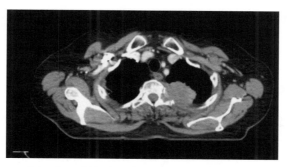

Fig. 29.3 CT scan of the chest following chemotherapy, showing a reduction in the left upper zone mass.

6. What are the further management options for this patient?

There are two options. First, it would not be unreasonable to adopt a watch and wait policy with a further CT scan in 3–6 months' time, depending on the symptoms. Clearly, this would not be curative but may be a pragmatic decision between the clinician and the patient. The alternative would be to attempt surgical resection of the residual tumour, rib, and part of the vertebra. This requires a full surgical work-up, repeat PET scan and lung function studies, and a good performance status.

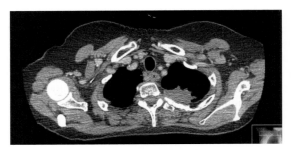

Fig. 29.4 CT chest scan following radical radiotherapy, showing a further reduction in the left upper lobe mass.

Follow-up and outcome

After discussion, the patient expressed a strong wish to proceed with surgery. She was referred to a thoracic centre for work-up for surgical resection of the residual tumour, first rib, and part of the thoracic vertebra by a combination of a thoracic surgeon and a spinal surgeon.

Repeat PET scan indicated negative lymph nodes and her lung function tests were satisfactory, therefore she underwent surgery. No residual viable cancer cells were found at resection. She had a complete response to chemoradiation and remained well 1 year from operation.

Further reading

Glassman LR, Hyman K. Pancoast tumor: a modern perspective on an old problem. Curr Opin Pulm Med. 2013 Jul;19(4):340–3.

Case 30

High-dose palliative radiotherapy

Kobika Sritharan and Julian Singer

Case history

A 64 year old male with a background of chronic obstructive airway disease (COAD), hypertension, and osteoarthritis, who was an active smoker with a 60 pack-year history, was seen in the respiratory clinic with a history of a few episodes of haemoptysis, shortness of breath, and weight loss. His ECOG performance status was 3. He was short of breath at rest but said that this was 'normal for him'.

Questions

1. What would be your differential diagnosis and how would you investigate this patient?
2. What does the CT image show and what are the next steps in this patient's management?
3. What treatment would you advise and how would you proceed?
4. What is the relevance of smoking and radiotherapy?
5. What possible toxicities will you consent for?
6. Comment on the CT chest scan findings and how you would manage this patient further?

Answers

1. What would be your differential diagnosis and how would you investigate this patient?

The differential diagnoses include lung malignancy, exacerbation of COAD, chest infection, and a pulmonary embolus. The patient will need a clinical review and a full history and examination should be carried out. He will need baseline blood tests and an arterial blood gas because he presents acutely with shortness of breath. He will also need a chest x-ray and a CT scan of his chest.

> **Case history continued**
>
> The patient had a chest x-ray and a CT scan of his chest (Fig. 30.1).

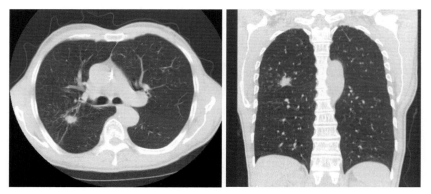

Fig. 30.1 CT chest scan of a smoker with a history of COPD presenting with haemoptysis and weight loss.

2. What does the CT image show and what are the next steps in this patient's management?

The CT image shows a 1.5 cm spiculated lung lesion in the right mid-zone. The patient should be discussed at the lung MDT meeting. He appears to have a solitary lesion on this scan and therefore the best method to obtain a tissue sample to establish a diagnosis should be discussed. As he is likely to go on and have some form of treatment such as surgery or radiotherapy, it is important to check his lung function tests as well.

Case history continued

The patient underwent a CT-guided biopsy. The MDT also decided to carry out a PET scan to look for any other potential sites of disease that were not seen on the CT scan. The CT-guided biopsy confirmed lung adenocarcinoma. His PET scan showed T1N1M0 disease. His lung function tests were: forced expiratory volume for 1 second (FEV$_1$) 620 mL, 21% of predicted; forced vital capacity (FVC) 740 mL, 19% predicted; and transfer factor of the lung for carbon monoxide (TLCO) 41%.

3. What treatment would you advise and how would you proceed?

The patient's lung function tests preclude surgery. Therefore he should be referred to the clinical oncologists for radiotherapy. If he had had a single solitary lesion he may have been a candidate for stereotactic ablative radiotherapy (SABR) despite his lung function. Unfortunately, owing to the presence of hilar nodal disease, this is not possible. He should be offered high-dose palliative radiotherapy for local control (Fig. 30.2) because of the poor baseline lung function tests and the high risk of developing long-term lung toxicities.

It is important to emphasize that he should stop smoking.

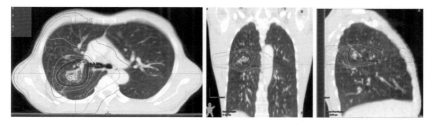

Fig. 30.2 Planning CT scan for high-dose radiotherapy for localized lung cancer.

4. What is the relevance of smoking and radiotherapy?

Smoking cigarettes or other forms of tobacco during the weeks a patient receives radiotherapy has been shown to reduce the overall treatment benefit. A significant decrease in locoregional control has been demonstrated in NSCLC.

Tumour oxygenation is important for achieving maximum efficacy from radiation treatment. The production of free radicals by radiation, which causes DNA damage and thus tumour cell death, is reduced with increasing tumour hypoxia. It is proposed that smoking tobacco increases the levels of carboxyhaemoglobin in the blood, which reduces the oxygen-carrying capacity of the blood. This leads to a reduction in the delivery of oxygen to the tumour and therefore reduced tumour kill by free radicals.

5. What possible toxicities will you consent for?

The patient should be informed about the potential acute and late toxicities of radio-therapy to the lung. The side effects of radiotherapy are determined not only by the anatomical location of the lesion, but also by factors such as the use of concurrent chemotherapy, prior surgery, proximity of sensitive normal tissue, total dose, dose per fraction, and patient predisposition.

Acute toxicities are usually due to an initial inflammatory reaction and are side effects that occur either during treatment or in the period immediately after. The pa-tient must be warned of skin irritation, including erythema, soreness, and dryness; oesophagitis, i.e. pain on swallowing or nausea; pneumonitis, i.e. increasing shortness of breath, cough, fever; and fatigue. He may lose the hair on his chest in the distribution of the radiation field.

Long-term toxicities are related to fibrosis of the irradiated tissue. Therefore, lung fibrosis, particularly in the context of poor lung function, should be mentioned. The patient is unlikely to get a significant amount of the dose to the spinal cord or heart but these are important areas to consider in terms of long-term toxicities. In the case of a Pancoast tumour, brachial plexopathy and shoulder stiffness must be considered. A secondary malignancy is a rare side effect but should be mentioned.

Case history continued

A year later the patient complained of increasing shortness of breath and chest pain after eating. He had a CT chest scan (Fig. 30.3).

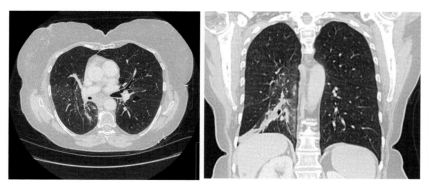

Fig. 30.3 CT chest scan a year after radiotherapy.

6. Comment on the CT chest scan findings and how you would manage this patient further?

The CT scan shows localized thickening of the interlobular septa in the right lower lobe. This is non-nodular and extends to involve the interlobular septa of the right upper lobe. This is likely to be radiation fibrosis and is within the radiation field. High-dose steroids may give some symptom relief. It is important to consider early lymphangitis carcinomatosis.

Chest pain after eating is likely to represent chronic oesophagitis. The patient should be on a PPI and referral should be made to the gastroenterology team for an endoscopy to rule out other causes.

Further reading

Baker S, Dahele M, Lagerwaard FJ, Senan S. A critical review of recent developments in radiotherapy for non-small cell lung cancer. Radiat Oncol. 2016 Sep;11(1):115.

Case 31

Stereotactic radiotherapy

Kobika Sritharan and Julian Singer

Case history

An 88 year old male had a stage I (T2N0M0) left upper lobe lung cancer resected 2 years previously. His past medical history included chronic obstructive pulmonary disease, hypertension, hypercholesterolaemia, myocardial infarction, coronary artery bypass graft, chronic kidney disease stage 3, chronic macrocytosis, and previous duodenal ulcerations requiring multiple laparotomies. He had an ECOG performance status of 2 and was able to walk at most 20 metres on a flat surface, limited by his breathing.

As part of his work-up for a recent change in bowel habit and abdominal pain he had a CT colonogram, which incidentally showed subpleural nodules in the left lower lobe. He had a thoracic CT scan to complete his staging (Fig. 31.1).

Questions

1. What does the CT scan of the chest show?
2. How would you proceed?
3. What are the treatment options?
4. What are the advantages of SABR?
5. What is the pathway to delivering SABR?
6. Who can be referred for SABR to lung lesions?
7. How would you follow up this patient?

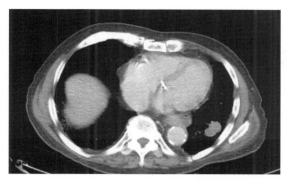

Fig. 31.1 CT chest scan showing an incidental left lower lobe nodule.

Answers

1. What does the CT scan of the chest show?

The axial CT image of the patient's lungs shows a 29 × 19 mm lobulated soft tissue nodule in the left lower lobe laterally. There are no enlarged hilar or mediastinal lymph nodes and no other suspicious lesions. The left lobe nodule was thought radiologically to be most probably a new primary lung cancer.

2. How would you proceed?

The patient should be reviewed with a view to taking a history, including of his general health and wellbeing, and carrying out a full examination. His case should subsequently be discussed in an MDT meeting with the expertise of a radiologist, respiratory physician, and thoracic surgeon. It would be common practice to carry out a fludeoxyglucose (FDG) PET uptake scan to add weight to the belief that these nodules are malignant and to look for evidence of other disease. The larger nodule in the left lower lobe may be amenable to resection if it is the only site of disease—this would probably involve a completion pneumonectomy depending on the patient's fitness.

Pulmonary nodules present a diagnostic challenge. Calcification usually suggests a benign pathology, and if a pulmonary nodule has been stable for a long period it is also likely to be benign. Lung MDTs usually have local pathways on how to follow up and manage nodules.

Case history continued

The patient went on to have a PET scan. This showed a 3 cm intensely avid nodule with a maximum standardized uptake value (SUV_{max}) of 11.2 (Fig. 31.2a). It also a showed a 5 mm nodule in the right lower lobe posteriorly, with much less avidity—an SUV_{max} of 2.3 (Fig. 31.2b). No hilar or mediastinal lymph nodes were seen. No other suspicious lesions were seen.

3. What are the treatment options?

There are two separate lesions, one in each lung, therefore the patient has no curative surgical options. Complete resection is recommended whenever possible. Given his extensive past medical history and a borderline performance status surgery is not likely to be appropriate even if he did have resectable disease. This is often the case in elderly patients with multiple comorbidities.

SABR is the treatment of choice for peripherally located lesions if patients are unfit for surgery, as in this case. A systematic review of SABR found local control rates of >90%. This has improved survival in elderly patients and reduced the proportion

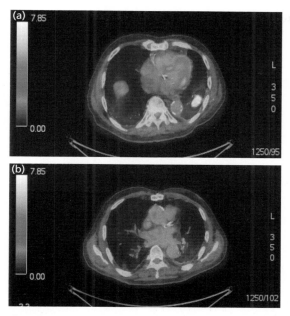

Fig. 31.2 PET-CT scan.

of untreated patients. Treating with SABR is also less intensive, usually with a total of three to eight treatments, than conventional fractionated radiotherapy, which is given daily for 5–6 weeks.

Alternatively, the patient could choose not to have any treatment as he is currently asymptomatic and has other ongoing medical comorbidities which are being treated.

4. What are the advantages of SABR?

Stereotactic ablative radiotherapy (SABR) also known as stereotactic body radio-therapy (SBRT), may be delivered by most modern linear accelerators or the Cyberknife system. SABR involves the use of multiple, highly focused radiation beams that are delivered from multiple points outside the body. They converge accurately at the tumour and are tailored to avoid radiosensitive organs that are close to the tumour. The culmination of these beams allows the delivery of high doses of radiation to the tumour. SABR is increasingly being used for patients with NSCLC who are not suitable for surgical resection and for patients who are unwilling to have surgery. The patient's disease was felt to be amenable to SABR.

SABR when compared with conventional radiotherapy is advantageous as it avoids the need to deliver high doses of radiotherapy to surrounding 'normal tissue' and reduces the overall volume of normal tissue irradiated. CyberKnife has a unique tumour tracking ability, including during respiratory motion, and has an accuracy of 1 mm. It also has an extremely sharp dose fall-off at the target volume margin when compared with conventional radiotherapy. This allows a much larger dose to be delivered to the tumour with significantly lower doses to surrounding structures. It is painless and non-invasive.

Case history continued

As the patient's lung function tests were satisfactory he went on to have 55 Gy/5 fractions using a CyberKnife platform to deliver the high-dose ablative radiotherapy (Fig. 31.3).

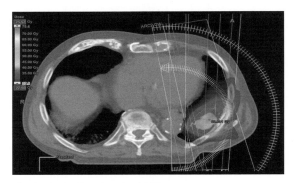

Fig. 31.3 CT planning for SABR.

5. What is the pathway to delivering SABR?

Oncology departments that are licensed to deliver SABR usually have a dedicated MDT to discuss patients' eligibility for treatment with SABR. The first step following this is a high-quality CT for careful identification of the target. A planning four-dimensional CT, incorporating tumour motion within the respiratory cycle, is then obtained in the replicable treatment position. The gross tumour volume (GTV), clinical target volume (CTV), and the internal target volume (ITV) are identified. The GTV is the macroscopic disease that can be visualized, and the ITV is the space occupied by the tumour during the whole respiratory cycle. The CTV is essentially the GTV in SABR. In conventional radiotherapy, a margin is usually applied to account for microscopic disease. These are encompassed to create a planning target volume.

The best plan is chosen when the decision is guided by dose–volume histograms. These allow doses for different structures to be compared. The radiation is then applied using a technology that tracks the tumour during the respiratory cycle following a trial run.

6. Who can be referred for SABR to lung lesions?

The UK SABR Consortium guidelines specify the following criteria for patient suitability for SABR in lung cancer:

- age ≥18 years
- NSCLC histology proven
- clinical stages T1/T2/T3N0M0 (<5 cm lesion)
- not suitable for surgery or patient refusal
- World Health Organization performance status 0–2
- peripheral tumours, outside of the 'exclusion zone', i.e. outside a 2 cm radius of the main airways and proximal tumours.

Patients who have had previous radiotherapy within the planning treatment volume who currently have more central tumours and in whom there is evidence of pulmonary fibrosis among other criteria are unable to receive SABR for lung cancer currently.

7. How would you follow up this patient?

It is recommended that patients are followed up 3 monthly for a clinical review for the first year, with 6 monthly staging CT scans for 3 years. In clinical practice, follow-up is usually tailored to the patient. Regular CT scans may not be appropriate if there are no suitable salvage treatment options.

Routine surveillance with FDG PET scans is not recommended because of a high proportion of false positive rates, but they may be useful in certain situations such as when recurrence is suspected based on a chest CT scan.

Further reading

Dahele M, Senan S. The role of stereotactic ablative radiotherapy for early-stage and oligometastatic non-small cell lung cancer: evidence for changing paradigms. Cancer Res Treat. 2011 Jun;**43**(2):75–82.

Murray P, Franks K, Hanna GG. A systematic review of outcomes following stereotactic ablative radiotherapy in the treatment of early-stage primary lung cancer. Br J Radiol. 2017 Mar;**90**(1071):20160732.

Vansteenkiste J, De Ruysscher D, Eberhardt WE, Lim E, Senan S, Felip E, Peters S; ESMO Guidelines Working Group. Early stage and locally advanced (non-metastatic) non-small cell lung cancer: ESMO Clinical Practice Guidelines. Ann Oncol. 2013 Oct;**24**(Suppl 6):vi89–vi98.

Section IV

Thoracic surgery

Case 32

A patient with T2N1M0 squamous cell carcinoma

Martin Hayward and Sofoklis Mitsos

Case history

A 64 year old male retired builder was referred to the respiratory outpatients department for review after his GP requested a chest x-ray. The patient's chronic daily cough of a teaspoonful of grey/white sputum for up to 40 years had now changed to include streaky haemoptysis. He had also lost 2 kg in weight over the last month, although he denied a change in bowel habit.

He was able to manage a flight of stairs and walk several miles on the flat without any problems. In terms of risk factors, he was a current heavy tobacco smoker with a 40 pack-year history and had probable occupational asbestos dust exposure for 10 years. There was no relevant family history of lung cancer, he was not diabetic and he was normocholesterolaemic and normotensive. He had moderate airflow obstruction on spirometry with a forced expiratory volume for 1 second (FEV_1) of 2.5 L (82%), a forced vital capacity of 4.95 L (86%) and a transfer factor of the lung for carbon monoxide (TLCO) of 62%.

The chest x-ray showed a 3.5 cm diameter mass overlying the right hilum with a small right pleural effusion (Fig. 32.1). CT scan confirmed a cavitating lesion of the right lower lobe with enlarged precarinal lymph nodes (Fig. 32.2). A CT-guided biopsy revealed squamous cell carcinoma (SCC) and a PET scan demonstrated that the lesion was fludeoxyglucose (FDG) avid with mild (just above the mediastinal blood pool) FDG uptake in the hilar and pre- and subcarinal nodes, and a non-avid pleural effusion and pleura (Fig. 32.3).

To more fully stage the subcarinal and precarinal (N2) nodes he underwent endobronchial ultrasound, which showed no evidence of malignancy in these nodes and that the preoperative stage was T2bN0/1M0. (The hilar N1 status was unknown at this time but had no bearing on a decision to operate on this patient since all these nodes are removed at resection.)

Questions

1. Would this patient be a suitable candidate for radical surgical intervention?
2. What procedures would be most suitable for this patient?
3. Is adjuvant chemotherapy beneficial for this patient with stage II disease?

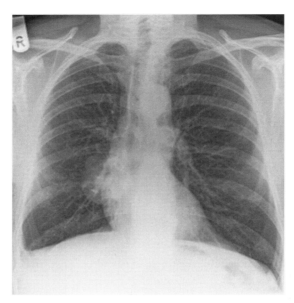

Fig. 32.1 Chest x-ray showed a right hilar mass with a small right pleural effusion.

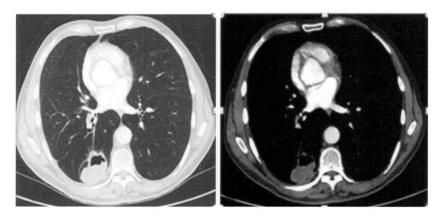

Fig. 32.2 CT scan demonstrated a cavitating 5.5 × 3.3 cm lesion of the right lower lobe with enlarged precarinal lymph nodes.

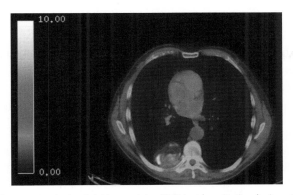

Fig. 32.3 PET scan revealed a right lower lobe FDG-avid cavitating lesion. Low-grade uptake of the small volume right hilar and right precarinal lymph nodes.

Answers

1. Would this patient be a suitable candidate for radical surgical intervention?

This patient has either stage IIA or stage IIB non-small-cell lung carcinoma (NSCLC) (depending on the hilar N1 status at surgery) with no evidence of metastatic spread. As such he was deemed suitable to consider for radical treatment by surgical intervention.

Surgery offers the best chance of cure for lung cancer but only 10% of patients in the UK with diagnosed lung cancer ever see a surgeon. The rest are either not fit enough or have too advanced disease at diagnosis. Surgical resection remains the primary and preferred approach to the treatment of stage I to IIIA NSCLC in patients whose performance status allows for general anaesthesia with single lung ventilation and a lung resection, as surgical resection in early stage disease is associated with improved survival compared with other treatment modalities. In general, the surgical removal of all stage II cancers results in over 25–30% of patients being alive with no evidence of recurring cancer within 5 years of treatment. At surgery every patient should have systematic mediastinal lymphadenectomy, which can be performed without increased morbidity. Surgery should be recommended in early stage lung cancer if a multidisciplinary team (MDT) and specifically a thoracic surgeon believes that the tumour is resectable and the risks of mortality and morbidity are acceptable to both the patient and his/her relatives.

The principles of management for early stage NSCLC

Complete resection is the goal of all operations for lung cancer. Proper diagnosis and staging are critical in determining the best treatment strategy for each individual patient. There are numerous non-invasive and invasive techniques that can be employed to establish an accurate and valid clinical estimate of tumour stage. If a contrast-enhanced CT scan reveals stage I, II, or IIIA disease, the patient should undergo PET scanning and mediastinal staging to exclude metastatic disease in those areas which would put him into stage IIIB or IV and make the patient either inoperable or unresectable. PET scanning is mandatory for all patients undergoing surgery and, in any case, is a useful baseline measure for the oncologist should the patient undergo chemoradiation as a treatment option.

Following confirmation that the tumour is *resectable*, the patient should be assessed for *operability* by assessing cardiac and pulmonary status and taking a detailed history, especially of other cancers. Patients contemplating pneumonectomy should have an echocardiogram to determine right heart function and pulmonary artery pressure, and this can often be done at surgical bronchoscopy by transoesophageal echocardiography carried out by the growing number of anaesthetists skilled in this procedure, or separately in the cardiac laboratory. The possible extent of resection will dictate the overall risk of mortality, but no current risk model has been shown to predict accurately the real mortality risk for lung resection. Overall in the UK, in high-volume centres performing over 150 major lung resections per year, the 30 day mortality for pulmonary lobectomy is around 2% and for pneumonectomy is between 4% and 8%.

An experienced surgeon should be able to determine whether a patient is at the higher or lower end of this spectrum and counsel the patient and relatives accordingly. Patients with borderline lung function should be considered for a lesser resection if the tumour anatomy allows and the patient informed of the possible freedom from disease at 5 years each resection offers. The improvement in cure rates with adjuvant chemotherapy against the mortality risk of the treatment itself should also be discussed at this stage to prepare the patient to expect postoperative chemotherapy in any T2 lesion and above, regardless of the eventual lymph node status.

A preoperative tissue diagnosis is exceptionally useful to a surgeon since it obviates the need for a frozen section at operation before proceeding with major resection, thereby saving operative time and a prolonged single lung anaesthetic. If a tissue diagnosis is not made preoperatively, an operative biopsy is mandatory, particularly in high-risk patients and those who require an extended resection.

2. What procedures would be most suitable for this patient?

In the absence of other risk factors and with reasonable lung function and exercise capacity, the most suitable operation for this patient is a right lower lobectomy with lymph node sampling or clearance with a mortality of up to 2% and a possible cure rate at 5 years of between 30% and 50% (depending on the N1 status) with some improvement with adjuvant chemotherapy. When set against the grim outlook for these patients if no treatment or chemoradiation is offered, nearly all patients and their relatives opt for surgery, despite the risks. In addition to clearly spelling out and recording the mortality risks for these operations the surgeon should counsel the patient about possible complications including prolonged air leak (particularly in those with emphysema), postoperative chest infection, and possible medium- to long-term pain in some patients, and postoperative dyspnoea because of the more limited lung capacity.

Alternative treatments

Although not ideal the peripheral nature of this tumour would make a lesser, or parenchymal-sparing, resection possible—an anatomical segmental resection with the relevant draining lymphatics would be possible here, or even a large wedge resection, and could be considered if the patient had limited lung function. The 30 day mortality is lower in these patients, but recurrence rates higher than those who have lobectomy, and highest in those having a wedge resection. Interestingly there appears to be no significant survival benefit with lobectomy, despite the lower recurrence rate.

Patients with inoperable stage II disease could be offered radiotherapy with curative intent with or without concomitant chemotherapy. New techniques, such as stereotactic radiotherapy and ablative procedures, are being evaluated in early stage lung cancer and may represent an alternative to surgery in patients unfit for lung resection. Primary radiation therapy remains the primary curative intent approach for patients who refuse surgical resection or who are determined by an MDT to be inoperable. There is growing evidence that stereotactic body radiation therapy provides greater local control than standard radiation therapy for high-risk and medically inoperable patients with NSCLC. The role of ablative therapies in the treatment of high-risk patients with stage I NSCLC is evolving. Radiofrequency ablation, the most studied of the ablative modalities, has been used effectively in medically inoperable patients with small peripheral NSCLC who are clinical stage I.

Case history continued

The postoperative histology report showed moderate to poorly differentiated SCC, 50 mm in maximum diameter, completely resected with clear margins (R0 resection). The PET warm hilar nodes were positive for cancer, but all of the N2 stations from (inferiorly) station 9 up to the subcarinal and station 4 paratracheal nodes were negative. The final stage was therefore pT2aN1M0. He was discussed at the MDT meeting and it was recommended that he attend for a discussion with the oncologist and be offered adjuvant chemotherapy on the basis that the tumour was >4 cm with positive N1 nodes and that he was fit and well.

3. Is adjuvant chemotherapy beneficial for this patient with stage II disease?

Overall 30–60% of patients treated with surgery develop recurrence. Many of these are systemic, indicating that adjuvant treatment might be beneficial. Several studies have confirmed the benefit of adjuvant chemotherapy in stage II NSCLC. In patients with operable stage II NSCLC, the evidence supports the use of three or four cycles of cisplatin-based chemotherapy after surgery. The benefit of chemotherapy after surgery is also present in patients who receive radiotherapy as part of their locoregional treatment. Potential long-term side effects need to be considered when deciding on chemotherapy after surgery and the mortality set against the possible benefit. There is insufficient evidence to support adjuvant chemotherapy for patients with an Eastern Cooperative Oncology Group (ECOG) performance status of ≥2 and in patients with surgically resected stage I disease.

No benefit in improved operability rates has been demonstrated by using neoadjuvant chemotherapy but it may be considered for those patients whose surgery may be delayed.

There is strong evidence, based on an updated individual patient data meta-analysis, that the use of postoperative radiotherapy following complete resection of stage II NSCLC is detrimental, and associated with worse survival.

Surgical procedures including lung parenchymal sparing procedures for NSCLC

Pulmonary parenchymal resection spans the range from pneumonectomy, bilobectomy, lobectomy, sleeve lobectomy, and segmentectomy to wedge resection, depending on the volume of lung parenchyma resected. From a technical viewpoint, with respect to the pulmonary hilum, these can be divided into non-anatomical (wedge resections) and anatomical (all other) resections. The characteristic feature of anatomical resections is that the parenchymal extent of resection is determined by the bronchovascular anatomy of the lung. For segmentectomy and wedge resection, the term sublobar or limited resection is sometimes used.

Although some debate exists regarding the extent of resection required for long-term freedom from disease for stage I tumours, the options are less contentious for stage II disease. The frequent involvement of hilar lymph nodes in stage II disease mandates resection that encompasses the nodal basin of the tumour. Even without nodal involvement, the larger size of these tumours (>5 cm) and their aggressive features makes lung-sparing techniques more difficult and less advantageous.

Lobectomy has recently become the standard of care for stage I NSCLC since the prospective randomized trial conducted by the Lung Cancer Study Group in 2015. Limited pulmonary resection, including anatomical segmentectomy and non-anatomical wide wedge resections, was compared with lobectomy for stage IA lung cancer. The Lung Cancer Study Group found an increased risk for locoregional recurrence, a reduced 5 year survival rate, and no statistical evidence for the preservation of pulmonary function, and thereby disproved the speculation that sublobar resection had an outcome that was comparable to that of lobectomy. Many studies have retrospectively supported this result, and have indicated that lobectomy carries an overall and disease-free survival advantage when compared with sublobar resection. Consequently, sublobar resection should now be used only for resectable high-risk patients, but should still be offered where possible. A note of caution should be sounded here, however, as in many such comparable studies the sublobar resection groups involved were medically compromised because of significant comorbidities, and these differences may have contributed to the poorer survival outcomes associated with limited resections.

As a segment represents a true anatomical entity in the lung with its own blood supply, bronchus, and lymphatic drainage, segmentectomy can be regarded as an oncologically valid procedure in patients with small tumours strictly limited to a segment, in whom lung function precludes lobectomy.

Wedge resections are non-anatomical resections consisting of the surgical removal of the lung tumour with as wide a surgical margin as possible to minimize the risk of local recurrence. It is recognized that wedge resection does not constitute an adequate lung cancer operation in most patients with lung cancer, but this may represent an acceptable option in patients with poor pulmonary function.

Owing to improvements in CT imaging and the introduction of CT screening programmes, smaller and pathologically earlier lung cancers are being encountered more often in our daily practice. This has led to a resurgence of interest in sublobar resection for early stage NSCLC and more specifically the non-solid lesions referred to as ground-glass opacities. These newly established clinical entities may be candidates for limited pulmonary resection particularly as the pathobiological nature of such earlier lesions is becoming better understood. It is not surprising that the possibility of managing smaller, earlier lung cancers by sublobar resection has arisen.

If we wish to advocate sublobar resection for early stage lung cancer, it must offer some clinically significant advantage in comparison with lobectomy, and the preservation of pulmonary function is one such meaningful advantage. Theoretically, sublobar resection such as segmentectomy has an anatomically functional advantage over lobectomy, since some segments of lung parenchyma that would otherwise be removed by lobectomy can be preserved. However, it is unclear whether the functional advantage of segmentectomy is as great as its anatomical advantage over lobectomy, and this should be confirmed in a prospective study based on adequate postoperative follow-up pulmonary function data.

Randomized clinical trials with peripheral lung cancers ≤2 cm in diameter as the target lesions were begun in the USA (Cancer and Leukemia Group B (CALGB) 140503) and Japan (Japan Clinical Oncology Group (JCOG) 0802) at almost the same time. The JCOG0802/West Japan Oncology Group 4607L trial is a prospective, randomized, multi-institutional study that intends to compare the prognosis and postoperative pulmonary function between patients with NSCLC ≤2 cm in diameter who are undergoing either lobectomy or segmentectomy. In North America, a similar trial entitled CALGB140503 is also underway, in which prognosis and preservation of pulmonary function are being compared in lobectomy and sublobar resection (segmentectomy or wedge resection) in a non-inferiority study setting. Clinical data from randomized controlled trials will shed further light in this area of controversy in the coming years. If these trials demonstrate that lobectomy and sublobar resection have similar curative effects and that sublobar resection offers better pulmonary functional preservation, sublobar resection should take the place of a lobectomy as the standard of care for patients with very early stage NSCLC.

Learning points

- The first aim of clinical staging and assessment is to determine the patient's suitability for radical treatment (resectability and operability).
- At present, surgical resection with systematic mediastinal lymph node dissection remains the gold standard treatment for early stage lung cancer, although few patients (<10%) present at this stage.
- Lobectomy or greater resection remains the preferred approach for most tumours, but lesser resections should still be offered to those with limited lung function when anatomically possible.
- Limited resections for stage II disease should be reserved for high-risk patients who would not tolerate lobectomy because of significant comorbidities or insufficient cardiopulmonary reserve.
- Adjuvant chemotherapy for patients with stage II NSCLC is well established with the improvement in recurrence rate increasing with advancing stage, but this is also offset by the increasing recurrence rate after surgery with advancing stage.
- Radiotherapy remains an important treatment for patients who are inoperable or who refuse surgery.

Further reading

Aokage K, Yoshida J, Hishida T, Tsuboi M, Saji H, Okada M, Suzuki K, Watanabe S, Asamura H. Limited resection for early-stage non-small cell lung cancer as function-preserving radical surgery: a review. Jpn J Clin Oncol. 2017 Jan;**47**(1):7–11.

British Thoracic Society and the Society for Cardiothoracic Surgery in Great Britain and Ireland. Guidelines on the radical management of patients with lung cancer. Thorax. 2010 Oct;**65**(Suppl 3):iii1–27.

Cao C, Chandrakumar D, Gupta S, Yan TD, Tian DH. Could less be more? A systematic review and meta-analysis of sublobar resections versus lobectomy for non-small cell lung cancer according to patient selection. Lung Cancer. 2015 Aug;**89**(2):121–32.

Gilligan D et al. Preoperative chemotherapy in patients with resectable non-small cell lung cancer: results of the MRC LU22/NVALT 2/EORTC 08012 multicentre randomised trial and update of systematic review. Lancet. 2007 Jun;**369**(9577):1929–37.

Ginsberg RJ, Rubinstein LV. Randomized trial of lobectomy versus limited resection for T1 N0 non-small cell lung cancer. Ann Thorac Surg. 1995 Sep;**60**(3):615–23.

Howington JA, Blum MG, Chang AC, Balekian AA, Murthy SC. Treatment of stage I and II non-small cell lung cancer: Diagnosis and management of lung cancer, 3rd ed: American College of Chest Physicians evidence-based clinical practice guidelines. Chest. 2013 May;**143**(5 Suppl):e278S–313S.

Nakamura K, Saji H, Nakajima R, Okada M, Asamura H, Shibata T, Nakamura S, Tada H, Tsuboi M. A phase III randomized trial of lobectomy versus limited resection for small-sized peripheral non-small cell lung cancer (JCOG0802/WJOG4607L). Jpn J Clin Oncol 2010 Mar;**40**(3):271–4.

NSCLC Meta-analyses Collaborative Group et al. Adjuvant chemotherapy, with or without postoperative radiotherapy, in operable non-small-cell lung cancer: two meta-analyses of individual patient data. Lancet. 2010 Apr;**375**(9722):1267–77.

PORT Meta-analysis Trialists Group. Postoperative radiotherapy for non-small cell lung cancer. Cochrane Database Syst Rev. 2005 Apr;(2):CD002142.

Sakurai H, Asamura H. Sublobar resection for early-stage lung cancer. Transl Lung Cancer Res. 2014 Jun;**3**(3):164–72.

Case 33

Long-term complications of thoracotomy: chest wall paraesthesia and neuralgic chest pain

Martin Hayward and Sofoklis Mitsos

Case history

A 62 year old female was referred to a thoracic surgical department with a biopsy-proven adenocarcinoma of the left upper lobe of the lung and no evidence of lymph node involvement or distant metastases. Her preoperative FEV_1 was 1.1 L (58% of predicted) with a TLCO of 52% of predicted. As the patient had borderline pulmonary functions, assessment of the predicted postoperative lung function was performed. Eventually, she underwent a posterolateral thoracotomy and left upper lobectomy. The tumour was completely resected and lymph nodes were negative for malignancy. Postoperatively she suffered from pain in the thoracotomy wound radiating to the anterior chest wall and was discharged home on oral painkillers. Ten months after the procedure, despite treatments with oral gabapentin and opioids, she was still complaining of post-thoracotomy thoracic pain. Resection of the affected intercostal nerves was offered with excellent results.

Questions

1. What are the methods for prediction of postoperative lung function?
2. What is the definition of postoperative thoracic pain?
3. Is there a surgical option for chronic post-thoracotomy thoracic pain?

Answers

1. What are the methods for prediction of postoperative lung function?

The surgical procedure depends on the stage of lung cancer and on the cardiopulmonary reserve of the patient. Medical operability of lung cancer has been frequently determined based on preoperative FEV_1, diffusing capacity for CO (DLCO), and the measured maximum rate of oxygen consumption which remains unchanged during a staged increase in incremental exercise (VO_2max); for the prediction of postoperative remnant lung function the anatomy of the lung must be understood. The right upper lobe consists of three segments, the right middle lobe two segments, and the right lower lobe five segments. The left lung is regarded to have nine segments in terms of volume: four segments in the left upper lobe and five segments in the left lower lobe. Each segment is assumed to have the same volume (1/19 of the lung function).

The four validated methods to predict postoperative lung function are as follows.

1. *Anatomical calculation.* Estimation of predicted postoperative lung function based on an anatomical calculation alone is simple, but the accuracy is slightly lower than other methods. Predicted postoperative FEV_1 ($ppoFEV_1$) can be calculated by subtraction of the FEV_1 proportion of resected lung segments from the total preoperative FEV_1.

   $$ppoFEV_1 = preoperative\ FEV_1 \times [1 - (number\ of\ segments\ to\ be\ resected/19)]$$

2. *Split radionuclide perfusion scanning.* The functional contribution of resected (right or left) lung is determined by the quantitative perfusion lung scan. Postoperative lung function is then estimated to be the product of the preoperative function and the portion of lung function that will remain after resection, as estimated by the scan.

   $$ppoFEV_1 = preoperative\ FEV_1 \times [1 - functional\ fraction\ of\ the\ resected\ lung$$
   $$\times\ (number\ of\ segments\ to\ be\ resected/total\ segments\ of\ that\ lung)]$$

3. *Quantitative CT scanning.* The basic concept is similar to the radionuclide perfusion scanning method. This measures the split lung function using the CT attenuation density instead of the radionuclide signal intensity. The volume of lung with attenuation between -500 and -910 Hounsfield units is used to estimate functional lung volume. The portion of the lung remaining post resection is predicted by calculating the lung volume in the area to be resected as a portion of the total lung volume.

4. *Dynamic perfusion MRI.* A study showed that magnetic resonance perfusion imaging had almost the same sensitivity and specificity for diagnosis of pulmonary perfusion defects as conventional perfusion scintigraphy.

The accuracy of postoperative lung function is affected not only by the calculation technique but also by the clinical factors associated with the anatomy of the disease—as mentioned earlier, a large tumour may occupy one or more whole segments, reducing the denominator from 19 functional segments to 18 or 17. Distal tumour consolidation may remove further functional segments from the calculation, and shunting through these segments may result in better oxygenation of the pulmonary venous blood once the shunt is removed. Finally, the resection of emphysematous segments in patients with chronic obstructive pulmonary disease (COPD), particularly with upper lobectomy, may produce a beneficial 'lung volume reduction effect', which again improves pulmonary capacity post resection. There will also be patients with central tumours who have 'autopneumonectomized' themselves prior to surgery or 'autolobectomized' themselves before resection. Experienced surgeons will take all of these factors into account when taking on patients with borderline lung function—a skill which takes many years to learn and borders on practising the 'art' of medicine alongside the science.

The actual lung function closely relates to the physiology of lung volume reduction, reversibility of airway obstruction, pharmacotherapy, and postoperative respiratory rehabilitation. A functional assessment (6 minute walk, stair climbing, and a cardiopulmonary exercise testing (CPET)) rather than static lung function tests are a more useful guide to operability in patients with COPD.

2. What is the definition of postoperative thoracic pain?

According to the International Association of Pain, the post-thoracotomy pain syndrome is defined as the recurrence or persistence of pain more than 2 months after thoracotomy, without any recurrence of disease.

Postoperative pain after thoracic surgery is particularly intense and prolonged when compared with other surgical procedures; different reasons may be responsible, such as rib spreading, costochondral dislocation, muscle division, use of diathermy, pleural trauma, pleural drain placement causing damage or inflammation to the intercostal bundle, and subsequent neuroma formation.

3. Is there a surgical option for chronic post-thoracotomy thoracic pain?

Efforts to reduce the pain of open thoracotomy incisions have led to the development of minimally invasive approaches to lung resection and other thoracic surgical procedures, as illustrated here. One option is to perform the surgery through closed ports inserted into the chest and with CO_2 insufflation as in laparascopic surgery. A surgeon trained in the use of a Da Vinci robot operates remotely while the experienced assistant remains scrubbed at the patient's side to manipulate swabs and staple devices (Fig. 33.1). The entire operation is carried out through closed ports with no rib spreading.

Another option is to perform lobectomy by means of video-assisted thoracoscopic surgery (VATS) carried out through a small non-rib-spreading incision with one or two additional ports as needed, and without CO2 insufflation.

Patients with chronic postoperative intercostal neuralgia not responding to medical treatment can potentially be candidates for surgical neurectomy. The site of

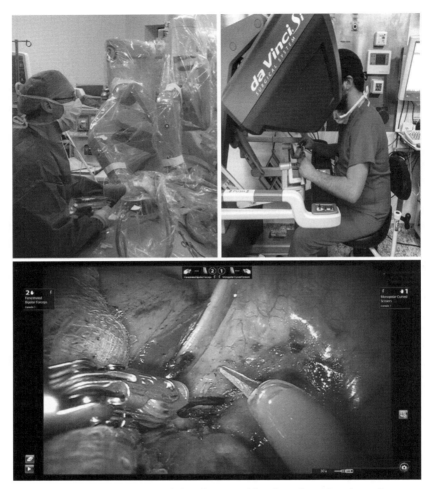

Fig. 33.1 Robotic instruments with five degrees of freedom dissecting the main pulmonary artery prior to closed robotic lobectomy.

resection depends on the location of the patient's symptoms and the known anatomy of these nerves; if symptoms follow a dermatomal pattern but there is no motor weakness, it may be possible to spare the motor portion of the intercostal nerve by resecting only the perforating lateral cutaneous branch. If the motor function is affected then the entire intercostal nerve may be resected proximal to the lesion. For patients who fail to improve after resection of intercostal nerves, there is still the possibility of performing a dorsal gangliectomy.

Learning points

- ppoFEV$_1$ is the most helpful indicator that a safe operation is possible as it provides fundamental information about underlying lung function and disease status. It has to be interpreted in the light of the patient's anatomy by experienced surgeons.

- A substantial gap is still present between ppoFEV$_1$ and the actual postoperative FEV$_1$, mainly in COPD and lung volume reduction surgery. This inaccuracy is critical in patients with marginal lung function following lung surgery.

- Moderate to severe COPD should not hinder curative resection of lung cancer if careful selection of the candidates is performed.

Further reading

Beckles MA, Spiro SG, Colice GL, Rudd RM. The physiologic evaluation of patients with lung cancer being considered for resectional surgery. Chest. 2003 Jan;**123**(1 Suppl):105S–114S.

Bolliger CT, Jordan P, Solèr M, Stulz P, Tamm M, Wyser C, Gonon M, Perruchoud AP. Pulmonary function and exercise capacity after lung resection. Eur Respir J. 1996 Mar;**9**(3):415–21.

Celli BR. What is the value of preoperative pulmonary function testing? Med Clin North Am. 1993 Mar;**77**(2):309–25.

Colice GL, Shafazand S, Griffin JP, Keenan R, Bolliger CT; American College of Chest Physicians. Physiologic evaluation of the patient with lung cancer being considered for resectional surgery: ACCP evidenced-based clinical practice guidelines (2nd edition). Chest. 2007 Sep;**132**(3 Suppl):161S–177S.

Kearney DJ, Lee TH, Reilly JJ, DeCamp MM, Sugarbaker DJ. Assessment of operative risk in patients undergoing lung resection. Importance of predicted pulmonary function. Chest. 1994 Mar;**105**(3):753–9.

Left pneumonectomy in a 25 year old female with a carcinoid tumour

Martin Hayward and Nikolaos Panagiotopoulos

Case history

A 25 year old Caucasian female was referred to an accident and emergency department after an episode of major haemoptysis. She had been previously well with no significant medical history with the exception of an episode of shortness of breath 4 years before. She was not on any medication and there was no smoking history.

Chest x-ray revealed complete collapse of the left lung with significant mediastinal shift (Fig. 34.1). A CT scan confirmed a 6 × 2.6 cm well-defined and enhancing endobronchial mass causing complete occlusion of the left main bronchus (Fig. 34.2a) with associated left upper and lower lobe collapse and deviation of the trachea and mediastinal shift to the left (Fig. 34.2b). No significant thoracic lymphadenopathy or pleural effusion was identified.

The patient underwent a rigid and flexible bronchoscopy that confirmed an endobronchial mass 3 cm from the carina. Multiple biopsies were taken confirming the diagnosis of a carcinoid tumour. A left posterolateral thoracotomy and a left pneumonectomy with lymph node dissection were performed, ensuring clear bronchial margins. The final histology confirmed the diagnosis of a typical carcinoid fully resected with negative lymph nodes (stage T2bN1M0). The patient's postoperative period was uneventful and she was discharged home on day 3 in excellent clinical condition.

Questions

1. What is a carcinoid tumour?
2. What are the epidemiology and clinical manifestations of a carcinoid tumour?
3. What are the radiological findings of a carcinoid tumour?
4. What is the management of a carcinoid tumour?

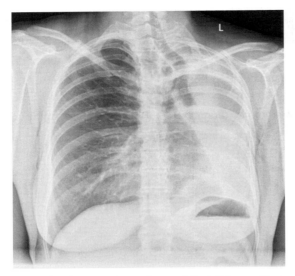

Fig. 34.1 Chest x-ray showing complete collapse of the left lung with significant mediastinal shift.

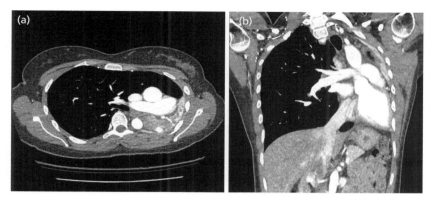

Fig. 34.2 CT scan showing (a) a 6 × 2.6 cm well-defined and enhancing endobronchial mass causing complete occlusion of the left main bronchus with (b) associated left upper and lower lobe collapse and deviation of the trachea and mediastinal shift to the left.

Answers

1. What is a carcinoid tumour?

A carcinoid tumour is a neuroendocrine (NET) tumour and is subclassified by the World Health Organization (WHO) into the following categories:

a. Well-differentiated carcinoid tumour (low grade, G1). This was previously known as a typical carcinoid and represents a benign indolent lesion that rarely metastasizes to locoregional lymph nodes (2–4%). No more than one mitosis is usually seen per high-powered field (HPF) and the overall 5 year survival reaches 100%.

b. Moderately differentiated carcinoid tumour (intermediate grade, G2), previously known as an 'atypical carcinoid'. The lesion presents with features suggestive of invasiveness but without invasion of the basement membrane. Between two and 20 mitoses are seen per HPF and the 5 year survival is 60–80%.

c. Poorly differentiated carcinoid tumour (high grade, G3). This is a malignant lesion invading the basement membrane, it metastasizes and is associated with worse prognosis. More than 20 mitoses are seen per HPF with features of degeneration, necrosis, and lymphovascular invasion. Overall 5 year survival ranges between 25% and 78%.

The G grade indicates the biological behaviour and aggressiveness of the carcinoid tumour.

Recently the Ki-67 propagation index has been described to help distinguish the grade of carcinoid tumour and is a prognostic factor for disease-free survival. Ki-67 is an antibody that adheres to the nuclear MKI67 protein that is required for mRNA transcription.

2. What are the epidemiology and clinical manifestations of a carcinoid tumour?

The most common location for a carcinoid tumour is the gastrointestinal tract, whereas bronchopulmonary carcinoid tumours represent only 10% of all carcinoid tumours. This is a rare lung tumour (1–2% of all lung tumours), with well-differentiated carcinoids occurring four times more frequently than moderately or poorly differentiated carcinoids. The peak ages of presentation are 40–50 years and they are mainly located centrally in a main, lobar, segmental, or subsegmental bronchus.

Symptoms depend on the location and size of the tumour and include the following.

◆ Cough, haemoptysis, recurrent chest infections, asthma, and unilateral wheeze as a result of airway obstruction or bronchiectasis. The first presentation may be sudden haemoptysis.

- The patient may be asymptomatic, especially with peripheral lesions presenting as an incidental finding.
- Paraneoplastic syndrome.
- Carcinoid syndrome, which is the result of serotonin secretion of the carcinoid tumour into the bloodstream. Symptoms include diarrhoea, palpitations, sleep disorders, dry skin flushing without sweating, and wheeze. It occurs in 2% of patients with bronchopulmonary carcinoid tumours.

3. What are the radiological findings of a carcinoid tumour?

- Chest x-ray: lung atelectasis, consolidation, bronchiectasis, and hyperinflation as a result of bronchial obstruction.
- Contrast-enhanced chest CT: this will define the location and relationship of the tumour with adjacent structures and possible lymph nodes and metastatic disease.
- PET scan: to confirm metabolic activity as evidence of malignancy. In a typical carcinoid the PET scan may not be active.
- Octreotide scan: the somatostatin analogue octreotide is used in the diagnosis of carcinoid and other NETs. Radionuclide scanning following intravenous injection of ^{111}In-octreotide (^{111}In-DTPA-pentetreotide) provides a sensitive, non-invasive method of localizing somatostatin-positive tumours.
- Bronchoscopy (flexible and rigid) and biopsy: for central carcinoids located in the main or lobar bronchi bronchoscopy can offer direct visualization of the tumour and multiple biopsies can be obtained. Carcinoids are extremely vascular structures and bleeding can occur during biopsy. For peripheral lesions in the lung parenchyma there is a role for CT-guided or surgical biopsy by VATS to confirm the diagnosis.

4. What is the management of a carcinoid tumour?

All carcinoids should be treated as malignancies and resection, even major resection if feasible, is indicated. Routine systematic lymph node dissection is an essential part of pulmonary resection for carcinoid tumours. Lymph node involvement is more common in patients with moderately or poorly differentiated carcinoid tumours, affecting long-term survival. Different approaches can be applied for the management of a carcinoid, as follows.

- Bronchoscopic laser resection: for entirely endobronchial well-differentiated carcinoid tumours.
- Lung parenchyma resection: depending on the location and size of the tumour a wedge resection, segmentectomy, lobectomy, bilobectomy, sleeve resection, or pneumonectomy can be performed to ensure complete resection of the lesion. Unlike NSCLC a classical carcinoid can be resected with a lung-sparing operation or lesser resection without compromising longer term survival because of

the non-metastasizing potential of these tumours. In this patient [and in several others at the authors' institution], the tumour was too central to avoid a pneumonectomy, but the 3 cm distance to the carina made pneumonectomy possible. Additionally this patient had already undergone 'autopneumonectomy', having entirely lost the function of the left lung before surgery—and therefore her preoperative lung function was already based entirely on one lung. It is possible that her functional status improved postoperatively because the surgery also eliminated any shunt that was occurring with pulmonary blood flow into the left lung in the absence of any ventilation.

◆ Chemotherapy: in patients with advanced local or metastatic carcinoid tumours cisplatin-based chemotherapy can be useful in 25% of cases.

◆ Radiotherapy: carcinoid tumours are resistant to radiotherapy.

◆ Octreotide (somatostatin analogue and somatostatin receptor antagonist): there is a role for octreotide in palliation of metastatic disease symptoms, failure of chemotherapy, and blood pressure control intraoperatively.

Learning points

◆ The majority of bronchopulmonary carcinoid tumours are located centrally (segmental, lobar, main bronchus).

◆ Depending on the size and location of the carcinoid a parenchyma-sparing lung resection is preferred, but major resection up to pneumonectomy is still an option with large central tumours.

◆ Radiotherapy is not indicated for the management of carcinoids and chemotherapy has a limited role.

◆ For moderately and poorly differentiated carcinoid tumours lymph node dissection is necessary and the nodal status affects long-term survival.

Further reading

Moore W, Freiberg E, Bishawi M, Halbreiner MS, Matthews R, Baram D, Bilfinger TV. FDG-PET imaging in patients with pulmonary carcinoid tumour. Clin Nucl Med. 2013 Jul;**38**(7):501–5.

Morandi U, Casali C, Rossi G. Bronchial typical carcinoid tumours. Semin Thorac Cardiovasc Surg. 2006 Fall;**18**(3):191–8.

Warren WH, Gould VE. Neuroendocrine tumours of the bronchopulmonary tract. A reappraisal of their classification after 20 years. Surg Clin North Am. 2002 Jun;**82**(3):525–40.

Warren WH, Welker M, Gattuso P. Well-differentiated neuroendocrine carcinomas: the spectrum of histologic subtypes and various clinical behaviours. Semin Thorac Cardiovasc Surg. 2006 Fall;**18**(3):199–205.

Case 35

Postoperative care of a 60 year old male with squamous cell carcinoma with severe COPD and no other comorbidities

Martin Hayward and Davide Patrini

Case history

A 60 year old male was referred to the respiratory outpatient department after an abnormal shadow on his left lung was identified during routine chest x-ray for his severe COPD. He could climb a flight of stairs and manage a mile walk each day. He stopped smoking 3 years previously but had a 50 pack-year history. He was on bronchodilators for his COPD. There was no relevant family history; his lung function tests showed a FEV_1 of 1.74 (67.5% of predicted) with a TLCO of 48% of predicted. To better assess the lesion a CT scan and then a PET scan were performed. These revealed the presence of a 4.25 cm left upper lobe lesion with a standardized uptake value (SUV) of 5. A CT-guided biopsy confirmed the lesion to be an SCC. After an MDT meeting discussion, the lesion was staged as T2N0Mx and a decision was made to perform a left upper lobectomy with systematic lymph node dissection. During the consultation it became apparent that the patient was concerned about his operation and recovery. He wanted to discuss the potential complications that can occur after the surgical procedure.

Question

1. What potential complications can occur after the above surgical procedure?

Answer

1. What potential complications can occur after the above surgical procedure?

The most common complications after lung resection surgery should be discussed and documented in the patient consent form—these would be postoperative bleeding, prolonged air leak, pain management, and chest infection. A general discussion about the need to mobilize, breathe deeply, cough, and mobilize the shoulder on the operated side should take place as well as a time line for the hospital stay so that the patient's and relatives' expectations can be put in place before admission. The median length of hospital stay for open lobectomy is 5 days, and for minimally invasive lobectomy by VATS or robot is usually 2–3 days only. Information on the need to place postoperative chest drains and their management should be touched on.

Postoperative management

Postoperative care of the thoracic surgical patient plays an important part in patient recovery and even survival and can be very challenging. Mortality after the index operation of lobectomy is directly linked to unit (rather than individual surgeon) volume and shows that experienced staff in high-volume units make a crucial difference to survival. Single surgeon volume is not correlated with mortality.

Thoracic surgery impairs postoperative respiratory function, resulting in a relatively high risk of developing postoperative pulmonary complications. The most frequent risk factors include age, poor preoperative pulmonary function tests, cardiovascular comorbidity, smoking status, and COPD. High-risk patients can be optimized with preoperative and postoperative cardiopulmonary rehabilitation to reduce their operative risk, frequency of complications, and hospital stay and to improve postoperative outcomes including postoperative lung function.

Pain management

Pain management is of paramount importance postoperatively as it is essential for patients to comply with chest physiotherapy and ambulation and they will not be able to do so if they have severe pain. There are various ways by which pain is managed. They include placing epidural catheters preoperatively, placing paravertebral blocks and catheters pre- or intraoperatively, or utilizing intravenous patient-controlled analgesia (PCA) in combination. On withdrawing these agents patients will need oral analgesics for a period of time until they are pain free. These include paracetamol, non-steroidal anti-inflammatory drugs and narcotic agents such as oromorph or oxynorm preparations. The resulting constipation these preparations inevitably produce requires the use of laxatives from an early stage to prevent straining and distressing constipation.

a. *Epidural analgesia.* Epidural local anaesthetics increase segmental bioavailability of opioids in the cerebrospinal fluid and increase the binding of opioids to m receptors and the blocking of the release of substance P in the substantia gelatinosa of the dorsal horn of the spinal cord. The thoracic segmental effects of local anaesthetic and opioid combinations are the only way to minimize motor and sympathetic blockade. They also allow conscious levels and a good cough reflex to be maintained and reliably produce increased analgesia with movement and increased respiratory function after thoracotomy. Generally the most popular regimens are fentanyl or diamorphine combined with levobupivacaine. Potential issues include failure, technical difficulty, and hypotension. Epidural analgesia can also reduce the effectiveness of coughing, especially in patients who already have a low FEV_1. It is not offered when there is local or systemic sepsis.

Paravertebral blockade is an effective way to provide pain relief. It can be done by the anaesthetist before the start of surgery or by the surgeon before closure. It offers several technical and clinical advantages and is indicated for anaesthesia and analgesia when the afferent pain input is predominantly unilateral from the chest and/or abdomen. This can also be combined with local blockade of the relevant intercostal nerves at surgery by the surgeon, and there is evidence to show that presurgery pain relief is more effective than postprocedure blockade. It is our practice to perform paravertebral blockade in the anaesthetic room and intercostal blockade in theatre at the start of surgery.

b. *Systemic analgesics.* Opioids remain the mainstay of postoperative analgesia and have demonstrable efficacy in the management of severe pain. The side effects include nausea, vomiting, ileus, biliary spasms, and respiratory depression. Opioids can be administered intramuscularly, subcutaneously, or intravenously. A very efficient method of delivery of opioids is via PCA devices. Numerous studies have demonstrated the safety and opioid-sparing effect of PCA. After thoracic surgery PCA is often combined with other modalities to offer adequate pain relief.

c. *Intrapleural local anaesthetics.* Intrapleural local anaesthetics produce a multi-level intercostal block. However, the analgesia is extremely dependent on patient position, infusion volume, and the type of surgery. With the drains in situ most of the anaesthetic is drained out and hence the efficacy of the procedure is reduced.

See Fig. 35.1.

Management of fluid electrolytes

Post thoracic surgery, especially after major resection, intravenous fluids are given in reduced amounts to prevent postoperative re-expansion pulmonary oedema and acute lung injury. Care is taken not to overhydrate the patient and oral feeding is encouraged as soon as possible. Intravenous fluids should be used judiciously and a conservative strategy of administration of maintenance fluids is recommended at 1–2 mL/kg/h in the intra- and postoperative periods and a positive 24 hour fluid balance of 1.5 L should not be exceeded. On the other hand, caution should be

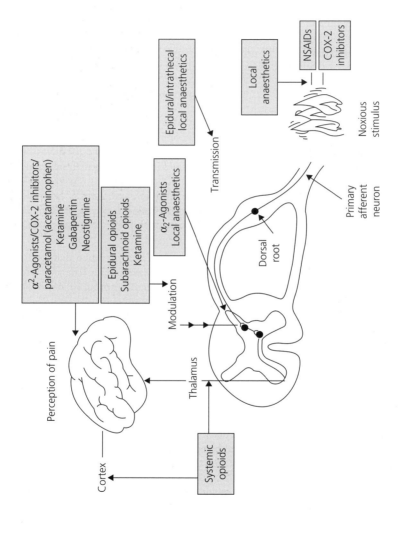

Fig. 35.1 Multimodal pain strategies. COX, cyclo-oxygenase; NSAID, non-steroidal anti-inflammatory drug. Reprinted from Pyati, S. & Gan, T.J. Perioperative Pain Management, *CNS Drugs* (2007) 21: 185 with permission from Springer.

exercised with regard to silent hypovolaemia, impaired oxygen delivery, and acute kidney injury. The postoperative team have to tread a judicious path between over- and underhydration in thoracic surgery.

Physiotherapy and early mobilization

Early postoperative ambulation and physiotherapy reduce complications such as atelectasis, pneumonia, empyema, and deep vein thrombosis. Postoperative pulmonary insufficiency may occur because of infection, the inability to clear secretions, or oedema around day 2 or 3. To prevent these from happening attention should be given to physiotherapy, bronchodilators, restriction of intravenous fluids, and tracheal toilet. Chest physiotherapy includes deep breathing and coughing exercises and incentive spirometry. Pulmonary insufficiency is more common in patients with a low FEV_1. Diuretics are used if necessary and antibiotics are started if clinically indicated without waiting for radiological deterioration.

Deep vein thrombosis prophylaxis

All thoracic surgical patients, and particularly those with cancer, should be given a prophylactic dose of heparin subcutaneously, if not contraindicated, at a dose 5000 IU once a day; this is continued in the postoperative period until discharge. All patients should wear thromboembolic deterrent stockings and signs of deep vein thrombosis should be investigated promptly by Doppler. These patients should receive a treatment dose of heparin by infusion.

Postoperative complications

a. *Postoperative haemorrhage.* Immediate postoperative bleeding can be due to surgical bleeding or coagulopathy. A set of standard coagulation tests are performed and coagulopathy is corrected accordingly. Depending on the coagulation profile, factors such as fresh-frozen plasma, platelets, cryoprecipitate, or factor 7 may be given. The threshold for taking back a patient for re-exploration should be low, as a surgical cause of bleeding should be ruled out. Bleeding after thoracic surgery is rare. It occurs in less than 2% of VATS procedures and around 1–3% of open procedures. A chest tube output of 1000 mL in 1 hour necessitates an immediate return to the operating room with concurrent correction of coagulopathy. Serial drainage exceeding 200 mL per hour for 2–4 hours after correction of a coagulopathy also indicates surgical bleeding and dictates re-exploration. If the patient is hemodynamically stable but the chest output is high, checking the haematocrit on the chest tube drainage can be helpful in distinguishing active bleeding from a lymphatic leak. If a patient in the immediate postoperative period is haemodynamically unstable but the chest tube output does not suggest active haemorrhage, a chest x-ray may show radio-opacity of the operated side with thrombosed chest tubes.

In the current era aspirin is a lifelong therapy and it is not necessary to stop it for surgery when there are specific indications for its use such as prophylaxis after stroke, acute coronary syndrome, myocardial infarction, or coronary revascularization, regardless of the time since the event that led to the recommendation of aspirin.

Dual antiplatelet therapy is seen more and more commonly in these patients, who frequently have cardiac as well as pulmonary problems due to their prolonged smoking habit and age range. These agents are given during the 2 weeks after simple dilatation, for 6 weeks after bare-metal coronary stent deployment, and for at least 12 months after the use of coronary drug-eluting stents. Because the majority of patients require surgery for malignancy and cannot be delayed then, unless the haemorrhagic risk is excessive, dual antiplatelet therapy should not be interrupted before surgery. Ticagrelor is used more often these days and should be stopped 36–48 hours prior to a planned procedure. Warfarin should be discontinued 3 days preoperatively, and the international normalized ratio checked. It should be substituted with heparin and the activated partial thromboplastin time checked.

In some patients, postoperative bleeding develops that is not haemodynamically significant enough to indicate re-exploration but results in a residual clotted haemothorax. As is true for a post-traumatic clotted haemothorax, treatment options include VATS or open exploration and evacuation of the haematoma to prevent development of a trapped lung, respiratory compromise, and empyema.

b. *Cardiac complications.* Arrhythmia, more particularly atrial fibrillation (AF), is by far the most common cardiac complication after thoracic surgery, with an incidence ranging from 10% to 20% after lobectomy and as much as 40% after pneumonectomy. Risk factors for tachyarrhythmias include those which are patient related (pre-existing cardiovascular disease, postural change, limited pulmonary reserve), surgery related (extensive procedure, intrapericardial pneumonectomy, extrapleural pneumonectomy, anaesthetic agents, major bleeding), treatment related (previous thoracic irradiation), or older age. The most common arrhythmia encountered is supraventricular tachycardia. If patients have AF with haemodynamic compromise then electrical cardioversion should be carried out immediately. If patients have symptomatic AF chemical cardioversion should be attempted initially followed by electrical cardioversion if necessary. New-onset postoperative AF is often transient and self-limiting and it is generally accepted that rate-controlling agents be given first. Rate control resolves AF in most cases in thoracic surgery. AF generally resolves within 1 day of hospital discharge with rate control alone. Amiodarone is not given if the patient has severe lung disease or if the patient has undergone a pneumonectomy, but some surgeons give prophylactic digoxin after all pneumonectomies with good effect.

Cardiac herniation is a rare complication and happens in the early postoperative period. Most documented cases of cardiac herniation have occurred through surgically created defects as a result of intrapericardial pneumonectomy or lobectomy with partial pericardectomy. Defects in the pericardium are usually repaired with Teflon strips, which may not prevent later herniation. Cardiovascular collapse is the presenting feature: the jugular pulse is elevated and there can be cyanosis in the drainage area of the superior vena cava. Ventricular fibrillation may occur.

Treatment is emergency thoracotomy with reposition of the herniated heart into the pericardial sac and repair of the defect in the pericardium.

Few studies have addressed the problem of postoperative right ventricular dysfunction, which occurs because of changes in right ventricular afterload and contractility. Although right ventricular end-diastolic volume remains stable in the early postoperative hours, significant increases may be observed on the first and second postoperative days. Changes in right ventricular function are able to compensate for the increased right ventricular end-diastolic volume at rest, but not during exercise, with a resultant increase in pulmonary artery pressure and pulmonary vascular resistance. Pneumonectomy patients have mild postoperative pulmonary hypertension without significant right ventricular systolic dysfunction. A proper preoperative assessment of right heart function and pulmonary artery pressure should preclude these patients from surgery and prevent this complication—it is almost impossible to treat if it occurs.

Pulmonary embolism and cardiac herniation are rare causes of right ventricular dysfunction which can be treated. Left heart failure is generally a consequence of impaired right heart function, either by decreasing left ventricular preload or by shifting the intraventricular septum, resulting in a decreased left ventricular volume.

c. *Postpneumonectomy syndrome.* Postpneumonectomy syndrome refers to bronchial compression occurring as a result of massive mediastinal shift following pneumonectomy. Incidence is approximately one in 640 cases. This syndrome is much more common after right pneumonectomy: the mediastinum undergoes counterclockwise rotation as it shifts towards the pneumonectomy space. This results in stretching, distortion, and compression of the left main bronchus between the pulmonary artery anteriorly and the aorta and vertebral column posteriorly. Patients typically present with exertional dyspnoea, stridor, and recurrent pulmonary infection within 1 year of pneumonectomy. The onset is usually gradual, but acute obstruction may occur in children. Definitive treatment involves surgical repositioning of the mediastinum in the midline. The mediastinum is then maintained in position by a saline-filled silicone prosthesis, which is inserted into the pneumonectomy space.

d. *Lobar torsion and gangrene.* Lobar torsion represents a rotation of the bronchovascular pedicle with resultant airway obstruction and vascular compromise. This disorder has been described in three different circumstances: as a complication of thoracic surgery, after blunt trauma, and spontaneously. The pathophysiological mechanisms of torsion development were previously postulated as an airless lobe, incision of the inferior pulmonary ligament, pleural effusion, a long slim lobar pedicle, and lack of pleural adhesions. The condition manifests as high fever, severe chest pain, massive haemoptysis, bronchorrhoea, and sepsis and is seen radiographically as abrupt consolidation and abnormal location of the collapsed lobe. Options for surgical intervention include simple detorsion or resection of the involved pulmonary segments. Detorsion alone is advocated only in patients who undergo reintervention within a few hours of the primary procedure, whereas, in the majority of patients, pulmonary resection is mandatory because of pulmonary gangrene. It is standard practice for some surgeons to staple or suture the middle lobe to the lower lobe after a right upper lobectomy if the oblique fissure is complete to prevent middle lobe torsion.

e. *Chylothorax.* The thoracic duct can be injured during any thoracic procedure. Pleuropulmonary procedures, oesophageal resection, intrapericardial and mediastinal procedures, and even less invasive procedures like subclavian puncture may lead to thoracic duct injury and subsequent chylothorax. Aetiologies in thoracic surgery include aggressive mediastinal lymph node dissection with incomplete ligation of lymphatic channels or direct injury to the thoracic duct during either extrapleural pneumonectomy or division of the pulmonary ligament. A prompt diagnosis and accurate early treatment are therefore essential. Analysis of the effusion demonstrates a triglyceride level >110 mg/dL and a lymphocyte count >90%. The total protein concentration in the effusion is near or equal to the plasma protein concentration. Conservative treatment initially involves replacing the nutrients lost in the chyle and draining large chylothoraces using a chest drain to ensure complete lung expansion. The aim of treatment then is to reduce the triglyceride reaching the thoracic duct either by keeping the patient nil by mouth and administering total parenteral nutrition intravenously or by using a diet containing only low-fat medium-chain triglycerides by mouth. Somatostatin and octreotide have proved useful as an adjunct in the conservative treatment of chylothorax. The success of this regime is evidenced by the pleural effluent into the drain becoming clear. The leak may then stop spontaneously as fibrosis occurs, and the patient is given a week for this to be achieved. If the leaks persists after this a return to theatre is usually needed to seal the leak, which frequently is difficult to find. Surgical therapy is also recommended in patients in whom, despite conservative management, more than 1.5 L/day in an adult or >100 mL/kg body weight per day in a child is drained, chyle at a rate of >1 L/day for 5 days is leaked, or there is a persistent chyle flow for more than 2 weeks. Thoracic duct ligation can be performed during thoracotomy or by thoracoscopic intervention, and in cases of loculated or complicated chylothorax pleural decortication with pleurodesis may be performed. Ligation of the duct is also usually accompanied by pleurodesis just to ensure the leak is properly sealed. Ward-based chemical pleurodesis with talc is an alternative option in patients who are too unwell for surgical closure of the chyle leak.

f. *Prolonged air leak.* One of the common problems after thoracic surgery is prolonged postoperative air leak, a complication that would certainly be discussed with this patient because of his emphysema. The Society of Thoracic Surgeons Thoracic Surgery Database defines prolonged air leak as lasting >5 days. Prolonged air leak may be associated with an increased complication rate and certainly may increase the length of stay in hospital.

By far the most common treatment of air leaks is watchful waiting with continuous drainage through a tube thoracostomy. More than 90% of air leaks seem to stop within a few weeks after operation with this form of management alone, with only rare development of an empyema. Patients can often be sent home with an indwelling drain attached to a Heimlich valve device or a valved bag system. The patient is managed through the outpatients department and the drain removed once the leak has stopped, assuming the lung remains expanded. There is no consensus on what the management should be if the patient has a prolonged air leak and a partially inflated lung or a pleural space after lung resection. Conservative approaches such as instilling autologous blood ('blood patch') or sclerosing materials into the pleural space through the thoracostomy tube may promote symphysis of visceral and parietal pleura and may produce leak closure, and the production of a raised diaphragm by creating a pneumoperitoneum may occasionally be effective, but many surgeons prefer to return the patient to theatre. Surgical options to accomplish pleural symphysis or control the source of an alveolar air leak, or both, include utilizing VATS with parenchymal stapling, chemical pleurodesis, and creation of a pleural tent or the application of topical sealants to the lung surface. Omental or muscle flaps placed at rethoracotomy can also be used successfully to obliterate the pleural space in patients with incomplete lung expansion and residual air leaks, but this is vanishingly rare. Most air leaks will seal as long as the residual lung and chest wall, pericardium, and diaphragm can become congruent, and this is usually achieved with judicial and careful control of suction on the pleural drains.

g. *Infection.* Infectious complications after pulmonary surgery include operative wound infection, empyema, and nosocomial pneumonia. Antibiotic prophylaxis should therefore be aimed at preventing these three entities. The incidence varies from 5% to 24.4%. Infections are responsible for increased hospital mortality to up to 19% as well as increased costs and length of hospital stay. Infections should be aggressively treated with appropriate antibiotics. Chest physiotherapy, pain control, bronchodilators, and early ambulation with a ward-based exercise regime should be the norm for all patients, but regardless of this pneumonia sometimes develops. Postoperative atelectasis after pulmonary surgery should be aggressively managed before it deteriorates into pneumonia. Early bronchoscopy to clear mucus plugs is extremely useful and in our institution the physiotherapist attends these sessions to help drive secretions into the bronchoscope by using vibration and manual techniques on the affected chest wall.

Empyema can develop if there is prolonged air leak and a pleural space with incomplete lung expansion. Generally patients are managed with antibiotics but empyema may necessitate thoracotomy and wash-out.

Postoperative care and the management of postoperative complications is a team approach and good preoperative and intraoperative measures minimize the incidence of complications; early recognition and treatment are essential for successful outcomes.

Further reading

Licker MJ, Widikker I, Robert J, Frey JG, Spiliopoulos A, Ellenberger C, Schweizer A, Tschopp JM. Operative mortality and respiratory complications after lung resection for cancer: impact of chronic obstructive pulmonary disease and time trends. Ann Thorac Surg. 2006 May;81(5):1830–7.

Scarci M, Solli P, Bedetti B. Enhanced recovery pathway for thoracic surgery in the UK. J Thorac Dis. 2016 Feb;8(Suppl 1):S78–83.

Stephan F, Boucheseiche S, Hollande J, Flahault A, Cheffi A, Bazelly B, Bonnet F. Pulmonary complications following lung resection: a comprehensive analysis of incidence and possible risk factors. Chest. 2000 Nov;118(5):1263–70.

Case 36

Preoperative assessment and fitness for surgery: T2N0M0 left hilar squamous cell carcinoma in a female with severe COPD

Martin Hayward and Davide Patrini

Case history

A 67 year old Caucasian female was referred to the respiratory outpatient department after an abnormal shadow on her left lung (Fig. 36.1) was identified on assessment for coronary angioplasty of a blocked right coronary artery. She also had peripheral vascular disease extending to her right superficial femoral artery. However, she could climb a flight of stairs and managed a mile walk each day. She had a glyceryl trinitrate spray but did not use this at all. She had stopped smoking 3 years previously but had a 50 pack-year history of smoking. She was on bronchodilators for COPD. There was no relevant family history; she was being treated for hypercholesterolaemia and hypertension. Because of a systolic murmur an echocardiogram was performed showing good left ventricular function and no evidence of valvulopathies. From a surgical perspective she had had a salivary gland removed many years ago. Her lung function tests showed an FEV_1 of 1.74 (70.5% of predicted) with a TLCO of 48% of predicted. To better assess the lesion a contrast-enhanced CT scan (Fig. 36.2 and a PET scan (Fig. 36.3) were performed. These revealed the presence of a 4.25 cm left upper lobe lesion with an SUV of 8.3 and no evidence of disease elsewhere either within or outside the chest. A CT-guided biopsy confirmed the lesion to be a SCC. After MDT discussion the lesion was staged as T2aN0Mx and a decision was made to perform a left upper lobectomy with systematic lymph node dissection.

Questions

1. Would this patient be a suitable candidate for radical surgical intervention and how would you assess her fitness for surgery?

2. What is CPET and what is its application?

3. How can preoperative functional status be optimized in patients with COPD before lung cancer surgery?

4. What is the difference between surgical techniques in postoperative complications?

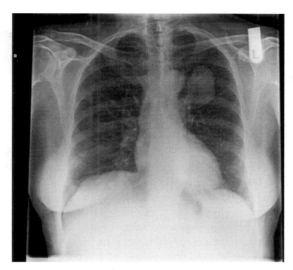

Fig. 36.1 Chest x-ray showing a left upper lobe shadow.

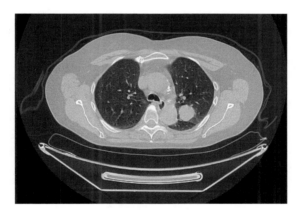

Fig. 36.2 CT scan showing a 4.25 cm left upper lobe lesion.

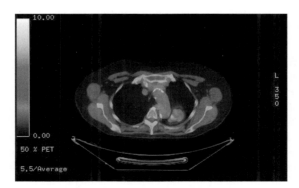

Fig. 36.3 PET scan revealed the lesion to be avid with no hilar/mediastinal lymph node involvement.

Answers

1. Would this patient be a suitable candidate for radical surgical intervention and how would you assess her fitness for surgery?

The scans indicate that this is a resectable lesion with the operation of choice being a left upper lobectomy, which would include the lingular lobe. The tumour involves no other structures and does not breach the fissure, and is clear of the lower lobe bronchus. A more limited resection is not possible in this case as the tumour is too central. Five segments of lung will be resected but one of these is almost entirely occupied by tumour, so any calculation of postoperative lung function would be based on removing four active segments from a total of 18, as opposed to five from 19. Since there is also an element of emphysema and the upper lobe is most affected, there will also be an element of lobar volume reduction effect, again resulting in a smaller reduction in lung function after surgery than in a patient with normal lungs.

The value of a preoperative assessment is to determine operability and to estimate the mortality and morbidity risk for this patient. The patient had already undergone an assessment with echocardiogram (to investigate the systolic murmur), which showed no evidence of valvulopathies, with preserved left and right ventricular function and, importantly, no evidence of pulmonary hypertension. A lung function test showed an FEV_1 of 1.74 L (70.5% of predicted) with a TLCO of 48% of predicted. Considering the lung function test result no other functional tests were performed as the patient was deemed suitable for surgical intervention on these results as well as her ability to walk a mile and climb a single flight of stairs.

An operable patient is someone who can tolerate the proposed resection with acceptable risk. It is imperative that the surgeon and the anaesthetist have a complete preoperative knowledge of the patient's medical status and also an appreciation of the pathophysiology of lung resection surgery.

For lung cancer surgery, the two prerequisites of resectability and operability must be fulfilled before pulmonary resection is even considered. Guidelines on the selection of patients with lung cancer for surgery, published by a joint working party of the British Thoracic Society and the Society of Cardiothoracic Surgeons of Great Britain and Northern Ireland, advise that fitness for surgery is based on an assessment of age, cardiovascular fitness, nutrition, performance status, and respiratory function.

Assessment of respiratory function and exercise capacity

It is strongly recommended that all patients who are candidates for surgical treatment of lung cancer should undergo both spirometry (FEV_1) and measurement of DLCO. As these two parameters represent the function of different lung compartments (FEV_1 is mainly associated with airflow limitation while DLCO describes the function of the alveolar capillary membrane), they are not strongly correlated. Preoperative FEV_1 and DLCO as well as calculated predicted postoperative lung function have been independently associated with morbidity and mortality rates in several studies. Some patients with COPD demonstrate only a slight loss or even an increase in respiratory function parameters after surgery, particularly with upper lobectomy, and this is attributed to the removal of emphysematous parenchyma around the tumour ('lobar volume reduction effect'). The decision to carry out surgery in patients with COPD should therefore be based mainly on exercise capacity tests rather that static lung function test measurements. As already mentioned, the size of a tumour may also mean that the removal of less functioning lung than otherwise would be the case will also affect postoperative lung function, and distal consolidation beyond a tumour may even have a third effect—that of reducing shunt through vascularized but non-aerated lung segments. All these effects are considered by thoracic surgeons, although the actual effect is almost impossible to quantify by any known test. Only a ventilation–perfusion scan might help estimate the size of any shunt, but its predictive value is unknown.

Thus the quantitative estimation of predicted postoperative lung function based on an anatomical calculation alone is the simplest but not the most accurate method. This, combined with the surgeon's experience of the functional anatomy mentioned above, is usually sufficient to determine operability in most cases.

ppoFEV$_1$ can be calculated by simple subtraction of the FEV$_1$ proportion or resected lung segments from the total preoperative FEV$_1$:

$$\text{ppoFEV}_1 = \text{preoperative FEV}_1 \times [1 - (\text{number of segments to be resected}/19)]$$

Patients with preoperative FEV$_1$ and DLCO >80% of predicted, or ppoFEV$_1$ and ppoDLCO >60%, are considered to be at low risk even for pneumonectomy. If both ppoFEV$_1$ and ppoDLCO are <60% then it is necessary to evaluate the patient's exercise capacity. This could be done either with low-cost tests (shuttle walk test, stair climbing) or with a CPET to assess the maximal oxygen consumption (VO$_2$max) as well as signs of ischaemic heart disease or heart failure. The shuttle walk test and stair climbing are strongly correlated with CPET. A cut-off point of 400 m for the former and 22 m (two flights of stairs) for the latter corresponds to a VO$_2$max >15mL/kg/min, which is considered adequate for performing lobectomy or segmentectomy. Patients with either ppoFEV$_1$ or ppoDLCO between 30% and 60% should be evaluated with low-cost exercise tests; if these are above the critical cut-off points then the planned resection is considered of acceptable risk.

The Thoracic Surgical Clinical Reference Group for the UK recommends that thoracic surgery should only be carried out in specialist surgical centres by experienced thoracic-trained surgeons and anaesthetists in specialist theatres with specially trained nursing staff. Thoracic units must have adequately trained and experienced recovery and intensive therapy unit staff, and the patients cared for in specialist wards by experienced and knowledgeable nurses. The surgery is inherently risky with patients who have multiple comorbidities, and minimum resection rates per year are required for a unit to function well and produce acceptable mortality statistics.

Cardiac complications are the second most common cause of perioperative morbidity and mortality in the thoracic surgical population. The commonest major cardiac complications are myocardial ischaemia/infarction and arrhythmias.

a. *Right ventricular function in thoracic surgery*. Preoperative evaluation of right ventricular function is not routinely recommended for lung resection in order to stratify postoperative complication risks, unless there is a suspicion of high baseline pulmonary artery pressure (PAP) or patients are scheduled for pneumonectomy. Ideally, the systolic PAP should not be >40 mmHg following surgery, and this has to be carefully considered if pneumonectomy, particularly right pneumonectomy, is being considered.

Advances in surgical and anaesthetic techniques have expanded the patient population that now qualifies for surgery. Preoperative assessment is an important step in the patient pathway to adjust the overall anaesthetic plan and customize monitoring to improve outcome. Several techniques are used to evaluate right ventricular function and PAP, such as two-dimensional echocardiography, tissue Doppler imaging, three-dimensional echocardiography, cardiac catheterization, and MRI. Owing to its ready availability transthoracic echocardiogram (TTE) is usually used as the first-line modality in the preoperative assessment of right ventricular anatomy and function despite its limitations (mainly related to right ventricular anatomy and the need for technical support). TEE finds its main role intraoperatively, especially in cases of pneumonectomy, extrapleural pneumonectomy, or lung transplantation, or in patients with significant parenchymal lung disease and baseline pulmonary hypertension. In the first two scenarios, in which the surgeon would want to perform a preoperative bronchoscopy, TTE can be carried out at the same time. Ligation of the main pulmonary artery can cause acute overload of the right heart, with dilatation and ischaemia or arrhythmias (occurring both intraoperatively and postoperatively). In patients with parenchymal lung disease, preoperative pulmonary hypertension may already be present and it can worsen during one-lung ventilation or clamping of the pulmonary artery. In these complicated cases, in which haemodynamic instability can occur during one-lung ventilation, echocardiography becomes a very useful non-invasive tool in guiding the extent of resection.

b. *Myocardial ischaemia.* Since the majority of patients undergoing pulmonary resection have a smoking history, they are at risk of coronary artery disease. Elective pulmonary resection surgery is regarded as an 'intermediate risk' procedure in terms of perioperative cardiac ischaemia. The overall documented incidence of post-thoracotomy ischaemia is 5% and peaks on day 2–3 postoperatively. Beyond the standard history, physical examination and electrocardiogram, further routine testing for cardiac disease does not appear to be cost-effective for all prethoracotomy patients. Patients with intermediate clinical predictors of increased cardiac risk (stable angina, diabetes, etc.) who have adequate functional capacity do not need further cardiac investigations prior to thoracic surgery. Patients with these intermediate predictors and poor functional capacity should have non-invasive testing of myocardial perfusion at rest and during stress with a stress echo. For patients who require coronary catheterization, the results may necessitate angioplasty with or without stenting or coronary artery bypass surgery before or at the same time as pulmonary surgery, but this is extremely rare.

c. *Arrhythmias.* Arrhythmias are a common complication of pulmonary resection surgery with an incidence of 30–50% in the first postoperative week if Holter monitoring is used. Of these arrhythmias, 60–70% are AF. Several factors correlate with an increased incidence of arrhythmias, including: extent of lung resection (pneumonectomy 60%, lobectomy 40%, non-resection thoracotomy 30%), intrapericardial dissection, blood loss, and age of the patient. Extrapleural pneumonectomy patients are a particularly high-risk group.

2. What is CPET and what is its application?

CPET provides an assessment of the integrative response to exercise of pulmonary, cardiovascular, haematopoietic, neuropsychological, and skeletal muscle systems, which are not adequately reflected through the measurement of individual organ systems. This non-invasive, dynamic physiological overview permits the evaluation of both submaximal and peak exercise responses, providing relevant information for clinical decision-making. CPET involves measurements of respiratory oxygen uptake (VO_2), carbon dioxide production (VCO_2), and ventilatory measures during a graded symptom limited exercise test. CPET is indicated for patients with limited lung function reserves on static measurement (ppoFEV$_1$ or ppoDLCO <30%). Patients with VO_2max >20mL/kg/min or 75% of predicted can undergo pneumonectomy safely, whereas those with VO_2 max <10–12 mL/kg/min or <35% of predicted represent a high-risk group and major anatomical resection is contraindicated. An intermediate risk group consists of patients with VO_2max = 10–15 mL/kg/min. In these cases an informed decision regarding operability should be taken with the patient in collaboration with the surgeon or alternative treatments should be discussed (wedge resection, stereotactic radiotherapy, radiofrequency ablation). CPET was not indicated in this patient.

Case history continued

Our patient had a 50 year history of smoking and she quit 6 weeks before surgery in an attempt to improve her mild shortness of breath. Because of her COPD the patient was on inhalers. Once surgery was confirmed the patient was advised to continue her bronchodilators to optimize her functional status before surgery.

3. How can preoperative functional status be optimized in patients with COPD before lung cancer surgery?

Preoperative functional status may be optimized with appropriate medical therapy, pulmonary rehabilitation, and smoking cessation. Although it seems logical that interventions, such as pulmonary rehabilitation, that improve COPD-specific functional scores (such as the body mass index/obstruction/dyspnoea/exercise index) might translate into improved perioperative morbidity and mortality, whether this is actually the case has not been tested in clinical studies.

a. *Medical therapy*. There is a paucity of data to demonstrate that medical optimization improves perioperative outcomes. Medical therapy for COPD can be maximized according to the guidelines set by the Global Initiative for Chronic Obstructive Lung Disease (GOLD) and the American Thoracic Society and the European Respiratory Society guidelines for COPD management. These guidelines include the use of bronchodilators (particularly long acting), often in combination with inhaled corticosteroids to manage the recurrent COPD exacerbations. Although it is possible that the use of oral steroids at the time of surgery is a marker for COPD severity or poorly controlled disease, the maximal reduction of systemic corticosteroid to a dose equivalent to 20 mg of prednisolone daily is appropriate in preparation for lung cancer surgery.

b. *Pulmonary rehabilitation*. A programme of rehabilitative exercise has been shown to improve exercise capacity in non-surgical patients with COPD. Such preoperative exercise can improve VO_2 sufficiently to move a patient from a physiologically unresectable category (maximal VO_2 <10 mg/kg/min) to a potentially resectable one. No definitive data exist to show that pulmonary rehabilitation alters short- or long-term outcome after lung cancer resection. A study of 22 patients with lung cancer and COPD, and who underwent lobectomy, examined postoperative outcomes after 2 weeks of preoperative aggressive pulmonary exercise and chest physiotherapy. These patients had decreased rates of prolonged oxygen supplementation and need for tracheotomy, as well as shorter postoperative hospital stays, than 60 historical control subjects who did not undergo rehabilitation. The study was limited to a single centre experience, small sample size, and use of historical control subjects. However, given the safety of pulmonary rehabilitation as well as its documented benefits in non-surgical patients with COPD, a recommendation of a pulmonary rehabilitation programme both before and after lung cancer resection seems appropriate in patients with moderate to severe COPD.

c. *Smoking cessation*. Many patients with COPD are active smokers at the time of cancer diagnosis. Given the relationship between smoking and respiratory complications in the postoperative period, smoking cessation has been proposed as a means of reducing perioperative risk. Pulmonary complications are lower in thoracic surgical patients who cease smoking for >4 weeks before surgery. Carboxyhaemoglobin concentration decreases if smoking is stopped >12 h. It is extremely important for patients to avoid smoking postoperatively. There is no rebound increase in pulmonary complications if patients stop for shorter (<8 weeks) periods before surgery. The balance of evidence suggests that thoracic surgical patients should be counselled to stop smoking and advised that the longer the period of cessation, the greater the risk reduction for postoperative pulmonary complications.

4. What is the difference between surgical techniques in postoperative complications?

The debilitating effects and the pain of a thoracotomy itself on chest wall function may well limit mobility and the ability to cough and breathe deeply after surgery, hindering recovery and possibly leading to postoperative consolidation and infection. In the last 10 years increasing numbers of surgeons have performed major lung resection by a minimally invasive approach, and the design and production of specialized stapling and cutting devices, energy dissection devices, and even specialized surgical instruments have allowed more patients to undergo VATS lobectomy using fewer and fewer ports. The original four or five port posterior approach has largely been superseded by a three, two, or even single (uniportal) anterior approach, and in the last few years a sub-xiphisternal approach has allowed surgery to be carried out without involving the ribs at all. There are now three centres in the UK where robotic lung resection through closed ports is being performed routinely, following the pioneering examples set in Italy, Germany, and France. Patients are mobile very quickly and usually home in 1 or 2 days, with a concomitant reduction in postoperative complications.

Although these approaches have shown a benefit in reduced length of stay and a reduction in immediate postoperative pain as well as equality in oncological outcomes, they have not shown any long-term benefit in terms of relief from longer term thoracic pain syndromes.

Learning points

- All patients having pulmonary resections should have a thorough preoperative assessment to confirm their fitness for surgery based on assessment of age, cardiovascular fitness, nutrition, performance status, and respiratory function.

- CPET is a global test of the cardiorespiratory capacity that reflects the entire oxygen transport system starting with the lungs and ending with the mitochondria. It is indicated for patients with limited lung function (ppoFEV$_1$ or ppoDLCO <30%).

- In patients with lung cancer and COPD, strict attention to quality of life becomes paramount. All patients should receive vigorous counselling regarding smoking cessation, both before and after a cancer diagnosis. Medical therapy of COPD should be optimized, with the intention of improving perioperative morbidity and enhancing quality of life. Attention to smoking cessation, pulmonary rehabilitation, and optimal medical therapy can maximize functional status, manage symptoms, and empower patients to take an active role in improving outcomes.

- Thoracic surgery is classed as a high-risk specialist activity and should only be carried out in specialist centres with sufficient numbers of cases annually to maintain acceptable mortality rates.

Further reading

Albouaini K, Egred M, Alahmar A, Wright DJ. Cardiopulmonary exercise testing and its application. Postgrad Med J. 2007 Nov;**83**(985):675–82.

Gould G, Pearce A. Assessment of suitability for lung resections. Contin Educ Anaesth Crit Care Pain. 2006;**6**(3):97–100.

Raviv A, Hawkins K, DeCamp M, Kalhan R. Lung cancer in chronic obstructive pulmonary disease. Am J Respir Crit Care Med. 2011 May;**183**(9):1138–46.

Section V

Palliative care

Case 37

An 84 year old female with advanced staged disease, dementia, and multiple comorbidities presenting with a suspected cancer diagnosis

Antke Hagena

Case history

An 84 year old female with mild dementia and multiple comorbidities was admitted from a nursing home for treatment of a chest infection. After a shadow was seen on the chest x-ray, a subsequent CT scan showed a left-sided lung lesion with lymph node metastases. The patient improved after treatment of the chest infection and was asymptomatic, but frail. She was able to mobilize with assistance of one. Her daughter was present to discuss further management.

Questions

1. Is a tissue diagnosis needed before one can discuss management?
2. Which options need to be discussed?
3. What is palliative care?
4. What assessment is needed to underpin the process of decision-making and patient consent?
5. What should the discharge planning cover?

Answers

1. Is a tissue diagnosis needed before one can discuss management?

No. On the contrary, the medical or oncology team should discuss the theoretical treatment options first, before making decisions about further investigations. If there is no subsequent treatment option, the benefit of interventions and investigations should be consciously considered.

2. Which options need to be discussed?

Ideally all treatment options should be explained when discussing a new diagnosis of cancer, and whether they are indicated, as follows.

a. *Palliative chemotherapy or immunotherapy*. Because of her World Health Organization (WHO) performance status of 3 the patient is unlikely to be fit for chemotherapy; it has to be explained that this is not a feasible option (Table 37.1).

Table 37.1 World Health Organization performance status

PS 0	Fully active, able to carry on all predisease performance without restriction
PS 1	Restricted in physically strenuous activity but ambulatory; able to carry out work of a light or sedentary nature
PS 2	Ambulatory, capable of all self-care but unable to carry out any work activities; up and about more than 50% of waking hours
PS 3	Capable of only limited self-care, confined to bed or chair more than 50% of waking hours
PS 4	Completely disabled, cannot carry on any self-care, totally confined to bed or chair

Adapted from Oken et al (1982) Toxicity and response criteria of the Eastern Cooperative Oncology Group, *Am. J. Clin. Oncol* 5(6):649–656 with permission from Lippincott-Raven Publishers

b. *Palliative radiotherapy*. This can be planned for symptom control or with an aim to prolong life. As the patient is currently asymptomatic, the indication would be to improve prognosis (benefit of months); any survival benefit should be discussed in comparison with the impact of a course of radiotherapy plus the preceding need for a biopsy and tissue diagnosis.

c. *Palliative care only*. This requires no further investigations. Treatment is based on symptom control and can be delivered in the community; palliative care is of course also available in combination with any palliative oncological treatment.

3. What is palliative care?

The *referral criteria* for specialist palliative care are:

◆ a progressive, advanced, life-limiting illness

◆ physical symptoms, or psycho-social or spiritual problems, that cannot be addressed by primary care or the treating team.

The modern model of palliative care advises a parallel approach with the disease-specific team; in this case, the oncology team. Some patients might never require specialist palliative care over the last years of life, others intermittently or continually, and others only towards the last months of their life. And while not all general patients require specialist palliative care input towards the end of life, most cancer patients should be referred because of the high incidence of symptoms.

Palliative care and end of life care are two distinct, but closely related, areas (Fig. 37.1). End of life care is defined by the National Institute for Health and Care Excellence (NICE) quality standard as care during the last year of life. Some patients will be identified earlier than others, and the level of input needed ranges from none over primary care only to integrated palliative care.

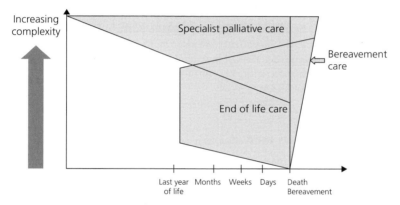

Fig. 37.1 Overlap between palliative and end of life care.

Early involvement of palliative care in metastatic lung cancer has shown positive outcomes for patients, better quality of life, less aggressive treatment at the end of life, a higher percentage of advance care planning discussions including 'do not attempt cardiopulmonary resuscitation' (DNACPR) decisions, and even a longer survival of patients (Temel et al. 2010).

Case history continued

During the discussion about the suspected new diagnosis of cancer, the patient appeared to have some short-term memory failure, but participated in the discussion. Her daughter was the patient's only relative and her next of kin, and both seemed to have a very close and caring relationship. The daughter asked whether it would not be easier if she made the decisions on behalf of her mother.

4. What assessment is needed to underpin the process of decision-making and patient consent?

The patient showed signs of memory impairment and has a diagnosis of dementia. But just because a patient has these conditions does not necessarily mean they lack the capacity to make a defined decision. This has to be assessed in this case in relation to the specific question of investigations and treatment for a suspected cancer and a possible treatment escalation plan.

The assessment and decision process is set out in the Mental Capacity Act 2005 (Box 37.1), which was designed to protect and empower individuals who may lack the mental capacity to make their own decisions about their care and treatment. It should then be documented on the hospital's agreed pro forma. Capacity has to be assumed and, if in doubt, all efforts must be made to support the patient to make an informed decision herself. Only if this is proven not to be possible, the medical team will have to make a 'best interest decision', taking into account the patient's previous wishes and ideas as represented by her next of kin.

However, it is important to consider that some patients prefer not to be given the full details of medical findings, diagnoses, and the possible future outlook. If this appears to be the case, ask the patient! Ask also whether the patient would prefer you to discuss the details with a person of their choice instead. Document this discussion in the medical notes, share with other professionals involved in the patient's care, and follow the decision made.

Case history continued

The patient was able to decide very clearly that she did not want to undergo further investigations or treatment. She was aware that her prognosis was limited to months, and that her increasing weakness was already a sign of the progressive cancer. She was keen not to stay in hospital for longer than needed and asked about discharge.

5. What should the discharge planning cover?

Ideally a *discharge meeting* should take place, inviting all people the patient identifies as important to her. This allows both the patient and her carers to ask questions and discuss any concerns related to the life-changing medical findings. It can allay fears and is the first step for an integrated handover to community services (Table 37.2).

The medical team has to consider the likely *prognosis*, even if the patient and family do not want to know, because it impacts on discharge options: hospices will generally admit patients for 'terminal care' if the expected prognosis is *short weeks*, usually 2 or 3 weeks (Box 37.2).

Box 37.1 Mental Capacity Act 2005

Principles

- Assume capacity unless proved otherwise
- Individuals must be given help to make a decision themselves
- Everyone has the right to make 'unwise' decisions
- When someone is judged not to have the capacity to make a specific decision (following assessment), that decision can be taken for them, but it must be in their best interest
- Treatment and care provided to someone who lacks capacity should be the least restrictive of their basic rights and freedoms possible, while still providing the required treatment and care

Two-stage Mental Capacity Act (MCA) test of capacity

I. Does the individual concerned have an impairment of, or a disturbance in the functioning of, their mind or brain, whether as a result of a condition, illness, or external factors such as alcohol or drug use?

II. Does the impairment or disturbance mean the individual is unable to make a specific decision when they need to? Individuals can lack capacity to make some decisions but have capacity to make the same decision at a later point in time. Where appropriate, individuals should be allowed to make a decision themselves.

A person is unable to make a decision if they cannot
1) **understand** the information relevant to the decision
2) **retain** that information
3) use or **weigh up** that information as part of the process of making the decision
4) **communicate** the above (by talking, using sign language, or through any other means)

Best Interest decision

If someone is found to lack the capacity to make a decision, and there is no advance decision to refuse treatment (ADRT) covering the decision and no lasting power of attorney appointed, the MCA states the decision must be made in their best interest.

Checklist:

- Encourage participation—do whatever is possible to permit or encourage the individual to take part
- Identify all relevant circumstances—what would the individual lacking capacity take into account if they were making the decision themselves?

- Find out the individual's views—including their past and present wishes and feelings, and any beliefs or values; review advance statements (not legally binding)
- Avoid discrimination—do not make assumptions on the basis of age, appearance, condition, or behaviour
- Assess whether the individual might regain capacity—if they might, could the decision be postponed?
- Ensure the presence of an independent advocate who will represent the patient's views—if the patient has no next of kin, refer to an independent mental capacity advisor (IMCA)

Data sourced from Department of Health (2005). *Mental Capacity Act.* London, HMSO under the Open Government License version 3.0.

Table 37.2 How to discuss prognosis—the *three don'ts*

Never disclose **uninvited**	Only discuss if asked, and ensure their question is unambiguous
Don't disclose **without warning**	Ask first 'What is your feeling?', then work from there
Never give **numbers**	Give prognosis as 'likely years/months/weeks/days/ hours', and acknowledge uncertainty

During the meeting the following areas should be covered, as far as appropriate:

a. Preferred place of care and preferred place of death—if the patient allows, this should be discussed sensibly but openly.

b. Current care needs—this does include the need for equipment or a package of care, based on assessments by the physiotherapy and occupational therapy teams. If a patient is living in a care or residential home, they will need to be assessed whether their future care needs can be met there.

c. Funding for care—if a patient has deteriorated rapidly because of an incurable disease, NHS continuing care will take over the funding, which—other than social services care—is not means tested.

d. District nurses—can be called out for emergency reviews, but the response time is usually hours, depending on the area.

e. Community palliative care team—refer if a patient is symptomatic or has other complex needs for end of life care.

f. Medication—if a patient is discharged for end of life care, 'just in case' anticipatory medication should be prescribed (see Case 40) and included in the take-home-medication, and the patient should be provided with a medication list explaining regular and pro re nata (PRN) medication.

Box 37.2 General referral criteria for palliative care services

Inpatient services

1. Hospice: admission criteria either
    *   symptom control (and discharge) or
    *   terminal care (if in the last 2–3 weeks of life)
    *   some units offer rehabilitation and/or respite admission
2. Hospital palliative care ward: admission criteria as above, fewer units in the UK

Community services

3. Community palliative care team: clinical nurse specialist-led teams with lo-cally varying multidisciplinary support at patient's home
4. Outpatient palliative care clinics: based at hospice units or in hospital, for patients who are mobile and can access outpatient services, often multi-disciplinary, sometimes offering specialist clinics (e.g. for neurological conditions, breathlessness, etc.)

---

g. Telephone list—the patient should also receive a list of telephone contact numbers and explanations of who to call when (community palliative care team, district nurse, GP, other services if indicated); failure to plan for deterioration or crisis will lead to distress and avoidable hospital admissions.

The discharging team should liaise with the nursing home, then inform the GP that the patient is being discharged back for end of life care. A GP home visit is recommended to sign a community DNACPR form, and then every 2 weeks for support, but also to enable the GP later to complete the death certificate.

Community services

Palliative care services
For general referral criteria, see Box 37.2.

District nursing services

Referral criteria either for regular nursing interventions (e.g. syringe driver assessment and refill, pressure area review) or for general palliative care (see the local policy for definition; can include monthly visits and discussion at GP Gold Standard Framework meetings). Normally there is a daytime service, and a twilight and night service; depending on geographic area, the usual response time for urgent call-out is 1 hour or more.

Carers

Funding

Apply in the patient's borough of residence.

Social services

◆ When people become frail and unable to care for themselves on their own, care can be organized by a social worker according to an agreed care plan. This will be funded by social services; the proportion of funding depends on means testing.

NHS continuing care

◆ If the need for care stems from a medical condition, and is complex, funding will be taken over by NHS continuing healthcare. The regular application process is based on a comprehensive *assessment tool*. All applications will be considered at the relevant borough's continuing care panel meetings, which usually take place weekly.

◆ If a patient is nearing the end of life, and has been rapidly deteriorating because of an incurable disease or health condition, NHS continuing care will accept a *fast track application* for funding. This requires a shorter application form and will usually be approved on the day of receipt. The NHS continuing healthcare team will then allocate a care agency to cover the required care plan for the patient at home, ideally within 24 hours or less, depending on the borough, or a nursing home placement.

Delivery of care

At home

◆ A *care agency* will be instructed by social services or continuing care to deliver an agreed care plan to meet the patient's care needs.

However, depending on the borough, the maximum care package available will vary: for example, from two carers visiting up to four times per day in some London boroughs versus a 24 hour live-in carer + a 12 hour night-time wake carer + four times daily double-up carer visits in the next London borough.

Depending on the maximum care package agreed by the funding authority, there might be local services to supplement care at home, for example.

◆ *Marie Curie night nurses* can be booked by district nurses or palliative care teams, and are either trained nurses or healthcare assistants. There might be a local limit to their use, e.g. only for the last short weeks of life, or only 2 or 3 nights/week.

◆ *Hospice at home* or similar services, where a hospice employs nurses and healthcare assistants to provide 24 hour care for patients at their home.

If the patient's care and medical symptom control needs become too complex, or if a patient states or had stated that their preferred place of death would be a hospice, he/she can be admitted after referral by either the GP or palliative care clinical nurse specialist.

Patients can also be transferred to a nursing home.

In a nursing home If a patient's care needs cannot be met at home or in their previous residential home, a nursing home might be suggested for care towards the end of life.

Nursing homes offer different levels of intervention, not all are able to provide syringe drivers, subcutaneous fluids, or intramuscular antibiotics.

The local palliative care team will support patients and staff at nursing homes.

Usually it is assumed that patients will remain at the nursing home for end of life care and would only be admitted to a hospice for complex symptom control problems.

Reference

Temel JS et al. Early palliative care of patients with mestastatic non-small-cell lung cancer. N Engl J Med. 2010;**363**:733–742.

Further reading

National Institute for Health and Care Excellence. End of Life Care for Adults. Quality Standard 13. London, UK: NICE; 2013. Available at https://www.nice.org.uk/guidance/qs13

Case 38

Titration of pain relief in a patient with right lung adenocarcinoma who received local radiotherapy

Antke Hagena

Case history

A 71 year old male patient who had previously been treated with local radiotherapy for an adenocarcinoma of the right lung returned to the lung clinic. He complained of a deep aching pain in his right back, which was radiating around his chest, in combination with spontaneous severe stabbing pains. Examination revealed bronchial breathing over the right posterior chest, and a painful tenderness in reaction to light touch over the area of pain.

Questions

1. Which term describes the abnormal sensation?
2. Does it indicate the underlying pain mechanism?
3. Starting and adjusting analgesia:
   a. What should be the first choice of medication to help with the pain?
   b. By what route would you give the medication?
   c. What do you need to discuss when consenting the patient, and which side effects do you have to mention?
4. Which other type of drug would you introduce next?
5. List two approaches to pain management that could be considered in this case, other than medication.

Answers

1. Which term describes the abnormal sensation?

Allodynia.

2. Does it indicate the underlying pain mechanism?

Pain in an area of abnormal or absent sensation is always *neuropathic* (Table 38.1).

Table 38.1 Mechanisms of pain in cancer and implications for treatment

Type of pain	Mechanism	Example	Response to opioids	Typical first-line treatment
Nociceptive	Stimulation of nerve endings			
Muscle spasm		Cramp	–	Skeletal muscle relaxant
Somatic		Soft tissue, bone pain	+/–	NSAID +/– opioid
Visceral		Liver pain	+/–	NSAID +/– opioid
Neuropathic				
Caused by compression				
Peripheral nerve	Stimulation of nervi nervorum	Brachial plexus compression by apical lung cancer	+/–	Corticosteroid + opioid
Central nervous system	Neural ischaemia (if prolonged = irreversible injury)	Spinal cord compression	+/–	Corticosteroid + opioid
Caused by nerve injury				
Peripheral nerve		Nerve infiltration, e.g. lumbosacral plexus	+/–	NSAID +/– opioid and/or TCA +/–anti-epileptic
Central nervous system		Thalamic metastasis	+/–	TCA +/–anti-epileptic

Reprinted from Twycross R. and Fairfield S. (1982) Pain in far-advanced cancer. *Pain* 14(3):303–310 with permission from Lippincott-Raven Publishers.

Case history continued

A CT showed a recurrent right posterior pulmonary mass invading the pleura and ribs, probably associated with intercostal nerve infiltration. The patient was already taking co-codamol 30/500 mg, two tablets four times daily, which was not controlling the pain. He had suffered a gastrointestinal bleed due to a gastric ulcer 5 weeks previously, and could not tolerate non-steroidal anti-inflammatory drugs (NSAIDs).

3. **Starting and adjusting analgesia:**
   a. **What should be the first choice of medication to help with the pain?**
   b. **By what route would you give the medication?**
   c. **What do you need to discuss when consenting the patient, and which side effects do you have to mention?**

Please see Box 38.1 for opioid guidance in palliative care.

a. For all severe cancer pains except isolated cramps the first-line analgesics are opioids. The first drug of choice should be *morphine*.

b. Strong opioids should be commenced *by mouth*, either with *regular* immediate-release morphine every 4 hours or with regular sustained-release morphine twice daily, and always combined with a *PRN immediate-release morphine* prescription to allow titration.

c. The patient's concerns and questions should be discussed. It is also necessary to address the impact on driving, explain the titration process, and alert the patient to the main side effects, namely

   ♦ constipation—prescribe a regular laxative

   ♦ nausea and vomiting—prescribe a PRN antiemetic

   ♦ drowsiness—mild drowsiness might resolve after the first few days; moderate to severe drowsiness indicates overdose, non-opioid-sensitive pain, or intolerance to the drug and the need for an opioid switch

   ♦ pruritus—allergic reaction: need to switch the opioid.

Case history

Over 4 days the sustained-release morphine dose was gradually titrated up to 50 mg twice daily plus 20 mg immediate-release morphine PRN. The patient was using three or four PRN doses per day, but described that, although the background pain had improved, the intermittent stabbing chest pains remained.

Box 38.1 NICE clinical guidance for opioids in palliative care

Communication and review

When offering pain treatment with strong opioids to a patient with advanced and progressive disease, ask them about concerns such as:

- addiction
- tolerance
- side effects
- fears that treatment implies the final stages of life.

Provide verbal and written information on strong opioid treatment to patients and carers, including the following:

- when and why strong opioids are used to treat pain
- how effective they are likely to be
- taking strong opioids for background and breakthrough pain, addressing:
  - how, when and how often to take strong opioids
  - how long pain relief should last
- side effects and signs of toxicity
- safe storage
- follow-up and further prescribing
- information on who to contact out of hours, particularly during initiation of treatment.

Offer patients access to frequent review of pain control and side effects.

Starting strong opioids—titrating the dose

- When starting treatment with strong opioids, offer patients with advanced and progressive disease regular oral modified-release or oral immediate-release morphine (depending on patient preference), with rescue doses of oral immediate-release morphine for breakthrough pain.
- For patients with no renal or hepatic comorbidities, offer a typical total daily starting dose schedule of 20–30 mg of oral morphine (for example, 10–15 mg oral modified-release morphine twice daily), plus 5 mg oral immediate-release morphine for rescue doses during the titration phase.
- Adjust the dose until a good balance exists between acceptable pain control and side effects. If this balance is not reached after a few dose adjustments, seek specialist advice. Offer patients frequent review, particularly in the titration phase (also see Communication and review).
- Seek specialist advice before prescribing strong opioids for patients with moderate to severe renal or hepatic impairment.

4. Which other type of drug would you introduce next?

Avoiding steroids shortly after a gastrointestinal bleed, the next step for neuropathic pain should be either an antidepressant, e.g. amitriptyline, or an antiepileptic, e.g. pregabalin or gabapentin (Box 38.2).

5. List two approaches to pain management that could be considered in this case, other than medication.

Oncological treatment or anaesthetic intervention could be considered.

Radiotherapy offers pain relief due to bone metastases, nerve compression, or soft tissue infiltration:

♦ Review previous treatment history and radiation doses to calculate whether the lifetime maximum tissue dose has been reached.

However, if the time since last treatment is only a few weeks, the disease is likely to be radioresistant.

♦ Radiotherapy is inappropriate if the patient's prognosis is very short (<2 weeks) as the response time is 3–4 weeks.

♦ A single dose is usually preferred over fractionated treatment.

Interventional techniques can also be used; for example, peripheral nerve block with a local anaesthetic and steroid. In this patient a block of one or several intercostal nerves would be appropriate.

Interventional pain control is an important option for a small number of cancer patients. These interventions can be delivered by anaesthetists in acute pain teams, interventional radiologists, and some trained palliative care physicians.

Box 38.2 Medication for neuropathic pain

First line

♦ Strong opioid and NSAID

Second line

♦ Step 1: Corticosteroid
♦ Step 2: Tricyclic antidepressant or antiepileptic, e.g. amitriptyline or pregabalin
♦ Step 3: Tricyclic antidepressant and antiepileptic
♦ Step 4: NMDA-receptor channel blocker, e.g. ketamine (specialist use only)
♦ Step 5: Spinal analgesia

Or else . . .

♦ As guided by the specialist team, e.g. alternative antidepressants and antiepileptics, topical lidocaine patches, methadone, benzodiazepines.

Interventional techniques include neural blockade and neurosurgery.
There are different types of neural blockade:

◆ Peripheral nerve block with local anaesthetic and a steroid, e.g. intercostal block.

◆ Sympathetic nerve plexus block with a neurolytic agent, e.g. coeliac plexus block for abdominal pain.

◆ Nerve root block with intrathecal phenol.

◆ Spinal anaesthesia with a local anaesthetic plus opioid.

Neurosurgery includes the following:

◆ Chordotomy, i.e. dissecting the spinothalamic tract, usually at the level of the cervical spine.

◆ Rhizotomy, i.e. dissecting a nerve root, usually in the lumbar region.

Further reading

National Institute for Health and Care Excellence. Palliative Care for Adults: Strong Opioids for Pain Relief. Clinical Guideline 140. London, UK: NICE; 2016. Available at https://www.nice.org.uk/guidance/cg140

Twycross RG, Wilcock A, Stark Toller C. Symptom Management in Advanced Cancer. Fourth edition; 2009. Nottingham, UK: Palliativedrugs.com Ltd.

Case 39

Management of cough, breathlessness, and haemoptysis for a patient who had previous treatment for small-cell lung cancer

Antke Hagena

Case history

A 58 year old female presented with cough, breathlessness, and haemoptysis. She had previously undergone a resection of a T1N0M0 right upper lobe small-cell lung cancer (SCLC).

Questions

1. Focusing initially on the breathlessness, which of the following treatments are available and what evidence supports them?
   a. oxygen
   b. opioids
   c. benzodiazepines
   d. steroids
   e. physiotherapy
   f. radiotherapy or chemotherapy/targeted therapy

2. Which medical treatments beyond the list above would you consider to treat the cough?

3. What treatment options are available for haemoptysis?

Answers

1. Focusing initially on the breathlessness, which of the following treatments are available and what evidence supports them?

    a. oxygen

    b. opioids

    c. benzodiazepines

    d. steroids

    e. physiotherapy

    f. radiotherapy or chemotherapy/targeted therapy

All are correct, and describe the collaborative work between oncologists and the palliative care team.

- Depending on the previous response to treatment and current performance status, the best option for medium-term control might be *anticancer treatment*.

- *Oxygen* has been proved to be beneficial only for patients who are hypoxaemic; therefore, it is crucial to check oxygen saturations at different levels of exertion.

- *Steroids* can improve bronchial or tracheal obstruction, superior vena cava obstruction, lymphangitis carcinomatosa, possibly reduce a malignant pericardial effusion, and have a role in patients with chronic obstructive pulmonary disease (COPD) or asthma. A treatment dose of, for example, dexamethasone would be 6–16 mg, depending on the severity of the obstruction.

- *Physiotherapy* has been shown to increase functional ability and thereby reduce breathlessness (COPD clinics will offer pulmonary rehabilitation based on this principle), but physiotherapists can also deliver breathing retraining and relaxation therapies, or airway clearance techniques.

- *Opioids* should be given ideally by mouth, either only *if needed* or *regular* (plus breakthrough doses). The starting dose can be lower than for treatment of pain.
  - For opioid-naive patients start with 1.25–2.5 mg oral immediate-release morphine. If a patient is already using opioids for pain, start initially with 50% of the analgesic breakthrough dose for breathlessness. Review and adjust: if needed reduce to 25% or increase to 100% or even more for severe breathlessness. While there is no evidence for the use of nebulized morphine, there is for oral and parenteral administration.

- *Benzodiazepines* have not been shown to have a specific antidyspnoea effect, but they play a role in treating anxiety and panic attacks.
  - Diazepam 2–5 mg twice daily and if needed is a starting dose, which can be increased stepwise. Avoid sedation unless the patient is suffering severe breathlessness during the last days or hours of life. In that case, and if the patient agrees, midazolam can be administered parenterally, as a subcutaneous stat dose of 2.5–5 mg. If this is needed more than once, start a continuous subcutaneous infusion (syringe driver) with a combination of an opioid

(morphine = first line) and midazolam to treat both breathlessness and agitation. Start midazolam at 10–20 mg/24 hours and review within the first 6–12 hours to ensure a dose increase can be prescribed if needed. It is not acceptable to leave a severely breathless patient to a slow titration of sedation over days. Involve the palliative care team for guidance.

Breathlessness is the individual experience of a breathing discomfort, and depends on physiological, psychological, social, and environmental factors that are often linked to physiological and behavioural responses. It is common among patients with advanced cancer, particularly for those with lung involvement, or can be caused by generalized muscle weakness.

A thorough history and physical examination remain the most important tools to evaluate a patient with dyspnoea, as no diagnostic test or biomarker correlates closely with changes in the subjective sensation of breathlessness. Common investigations include chest x-ray and full blood count; specific tests like ultrasound, CT pulmonary angiography, spirometry or peak flow, d-dimer, brain natriuretic peptide, and arterial blood gases have their diagnostic role in specific clinical circumstances.

If there is an underlying reversible cause, treatment should be optimized. Cancer-related causes can affect different systems, e.g. pleural or pericardial effusion or ascites. Equally cancer treatment can be the cause; examples are pulmonary fibrosis post radiotherapy or pneumonitis in reaction to chemotherapy, targeted drugs, or immunotherapies. Patients with cancer are at higher risk of developing comorbidities, such as pneumonia or pulmonary embolism. And, finally, there can be the range of further medical history, be it COPD, asthma, or heart failure.

Non-drug treatment involves *physiotherapists* for breathing *re-training*, or relaxation techniques and to maximize functional ability; *counsellors* or *psychologists* can offer support for coping with associated anxiety and the effect on the general and social quality of life, both for the patient and those close to her.

Complementary therapies might benefit some. There is also evidence that the use of an electric fan can decrease the sensation of breathlessness.

Drug treatment will consist of bronchodilators where indicated, e.g. a β2-adrenergic receptor stimulant combined, if needed, with an antimuscarinic via a spacer or nebulizer to reduce air trapping.

Opioids can relieve breathlessness by one or more different mechanisms: decreasing respiratory effort (associated decreased corollary discharge), altering central perception, altering the activity of peripheral opioid receptors in the lung, and by decreasing anxiety. This benefit of a decreased respiratory effort is evident at doses that do not cause respiratory depression.

Opioids work mostly for patients who are breathless at rest, as dyspnoea after exertion usually resolves within a few minutes, faster than the time to onset of an oral morphine preparation (20–30 minutes).

Although there is no evidence for the use of benzodiazepines to specifically treat shortness of breath, patients will often develop anxiety and panic attacks, which might then require the use of anxiolytic oxygen if needed.

Oxygen should be started if hypoxaemia is proven (S_aO_2 >90%). Studies seem to show that the combination of airflow and a cooling effect are responsible for the relieving effect in other patients. So an electric fan or open window should be tried first for patients with good oxygenation, before offering oxygen.

If a patient with severe breathlessness is using oxygen and finds it helpful, this should be continued.

Helium–oxygen mixtures have been used sporadically, but are limited because of cost and practical difficulties of transport, as each large cylinder lasts for only 2–3 hours.

2. Which medical treatments beyond the list above would you consider to treat the cough?

The first-line treatment are opioids to suppress the cough reflex.

As second-line treatment, if the cough is productive but the patient is unable to expectorate NaCl nebulizers and acetylcysteine should be used.

3. What treatment options are available for haemoptysis?

As the haemoptysis is currently not severe, this can first be treated conservatively:

◆ Stop medication that increases risk: low molecular weight heparin, warfarin, aspirin, NSAIDs

◆ If the platelet count is <30/L, consider a platelet transfusion. This will last for 7–10 days, so requires further advance care planning.

◆ If neither apply, or as next step start tranexamic acid 1 g three times daily orally or intravenously (Box 39.1).

Box 39.1 Tranexamic acid

Tranexamic acid is an antifibrinolytic drug that binds to plasminogen receptors, thereby preventing fibrin activation and consequent fibrinolysis.

Treatment should generally continue for 3 days after bleeding has stopped, and should be restarted if further bleeding develops. If continuing treatment is needed, doses can be from 500 mg three times daily and up to 1 g four times daily.

Other important treatment options would include a short course of radiotherapy, or bronchoscopy with laser coagulation.

The severity and prognosis should be considered when planning these treatments:

◆ Treat the accompanying anxiety with a benzodiazepine, e.g. lorazepam 0.5–1.0 mg sublingually or midazolam 2.5–5.0 mg subcutaneously.

- Herald bleed: even if haemoptysis is mild, preparation should be made for a possible major haemorrhage.

Sudden severe haemoptysis

Twenty per cent of patients with lung cancer will experience haemoptysis, which can be due to a direct tumour effect, thrombocytopenia, or side effects of treatment (e.g. bevacizumab). New onset mild haemoptysis is most likely to be due to superficial tumour bleeding.

An *acute fatal bleed* is a relatively rare event: 3% in one study, with a mortality of 59–100%. As it is unlikely to be amenable to interventional treatment, this should be included in planning the ceiling of care. If it happens, it is a frightening event for the patient, for visitors, and also for staff. Prepare with the following.

1. A dark blanket—to reduce the fear-inducing visibility of blood, it is recommended to have a dark-coloured blanket ready in the room; this can be used to cover white bedlinen or clothes to decrease the visibility of bright red blood.
2. A crisis pack—to reduce the patient's fear and possible pain or breathlessness, give a fast-acting parenteral (intravenous if access is established, intramuscularly otherwise) dose of benzodiazepine and opioid at double the current PRN dose, e.g.

    a. midazolam 10 mg intravenously/intramuscularly and
    b. morphine 10 mg (if the patient is not on opioids).

    In a terminal event accumulation is not relevant, so in general prescribe the patient's current opioid.

3. Nursing handover—This is most important to ensure quick reaction and awareness of the treatment aim, i.e. the patient's comfort.

Further reading

Clemens KE, Quednau I, Klaschik E. Is there a higher risk of respiratory depression in opioid-naïve palliative care patients during symptomatic therapy of dyspnea with strong opioids? J Palliat Med. 2008 Mar;**11**(2):204–16.

Jennings AL, Davies AN, Higgins JP, Gibbs JS, Broadley KE. A systematic review of the use of opioids in the management of dyspnea. Thorax. 2002 Nov;**57**(11):939–44.

Kvale PA, Simoff M, Prakash UB; American College of Chest Physicians. Lung cancer. Palliative care. Chest. 2003 Jan;**123**(1 Suppl):284S–311S.

Miller RR, McGregor DH. Hemorrhage from carcinoma of the lung. Cancer. 1980 Jul;**46**(1):200.

National Institute for Health and Care Excellence. Blood Transfusion. NICE Guideline 24. London, UK: NICE; 2015. Available at https://www.nice.org.uk/guidance/ng24/chapter/recommendations#platelets-2

Simon ST, Higginson IJ, Booth S, Harding R, Bausewein C. Benzodiazepines for the relief of breathlessness in advanced malignant and non-malignant diseases in adults. Cochrane Database Syst Rev. 2010 Jan;(1):CD007354.

Case 40

A former builder with pleural effusions secondary to mesothelioma

Antke Hagena

Case history

A 61 year old male builder presented with marked breathlessness. He had previously received palliative chemotherapy for an epithelial malignant mesothelioma. Now a chest x-ray showed a moderate left pleural effusion.

Questions

1. What information should you check with the patient from a sociolegal point of view?
2. What is the approximate amount of pleural fluid that can be routinely detected on a posteroanterior chest x-ray?
3. Does the presence of a pleural effusion affect the patient's prognosis?
4. Which factors will influence the decision-making of the multidisciplinary team (MDT) regarding further management of the pleural effusion?
5. What would be the maximum volume to drain during an initial pleural aspiration, and why?
6. Which options are available that would aim for a longer term solution than a simple thoracocentesis?
7. Is there any other recommendation post thoracoscopy, specifically for patients with mesothelioma?

Answers

1. What information should you check with the patient from a sociolegal point of view?

Clarify whether the patient has already been supported to submit a *compensation claim.*

◆ Most cases of mesothelioma are caused by asbestos exposure.

◆ An occupational history of exposure, e.g. builder, shipyard worker, entitles the patient to compensation payment.

◆ Clinical presentation is often 30–40 years after exposure.

The patient should contact a law firm experienced in dealing with mesothelioma compensation claims, which can be found easily by Internet search. The law firm will then lead the case and be aware of time limits and information needs. Beware that any death that may have resulted from an occupational disease has to be reported to the coroner.

2. What is the approximate amount of pleural fluid that can be routinely detected on a posteroanterior chest x-ray?

The posteroanterior chest x-ray will be abnormal with a volume of about 200 mL of pleural fluid. A lateral chest x-ray is more sensitive and will detect a volume of about 50 mL, evident from blunting of the posterior costophrenic angle. Clinical examination will rarely detect an effusion of <500 mL.

3. Does the presence of a pleural effusion affect the patient's prognosis?

Based on a number of studies the median survival following a new diagnosis of malignant pleural effusion ranges from 3 to 12 months; in newer studies, this is up to 15 months, depending on the underlying primary, and reflects developments in cancer treatment.

Case history continued

A CT scan confirmed a recurrent pleural mass and a moderately sized pleural effusion. This was assumed to be a recurrence of the mesothelioma.

4. Which factors will influence the decision-making of the MDT regarding further management of the pleural effusion?

If cytology confirms recurrent mesothelioma, further treatment will depend on the:

- likelihood of the cancer responding to further chemotherapy; this is less likely for mesothelioma, but more likely, for example, for SCLC, lymphoma, or breast cancer
- severity of symptoms: small asymptomatic effusions are best just monitored; symptomatic effusions should be drained
- degree of lung re-expansion after initial pleural fluid evacuation
- patient's performance status and prognosis.

5. What would be the maximum volume to drain during an initial pleural aspiration, and why?

The recommended maximum drainage volume is 1500 mL, at a rate of about 500 mL/h to avoid re-expansion pulmonary oedema. As 50% of malignant pleural effusions recur within 4 days, and 97% within 4 weeks, one should consider long-term options for patients with a prognosis >1 month.

6. Which options are available that would aim for a longer term solution than a simple thoracocentesis?

To reduce the risk of reaccumulation there are the following options:

1. *Video-assisted thoracoscopic surgery (VATS) pleurodesis* under sedation or general anaesthesia—for patients with a reasonable prognosis; talc installation with an atomizer (poudrage) acts as a sclerosant inducing inflammation and activation of the coagulation system with fibrin production; this prevents recurrence of effusions in >90%.

2. *Chest tube drainage and medical pleurodesis*—after re-expansion of the lung a lidocaine solution is instilled into the pleural space, followed by the sclerosant (= talc slurry); this achieves long-term control in >50%.

   Side effects of any pleurodesis procedure can be chest pain and fever. Steroids, both local and systemic, have been shown to impair the effectiveness of pleurodesis. Most studies have shown that lack of response to pleurodesis is associated with incomplete expansion of the lung, due to visceral thickening (trapped lung), loculated effusions, proximal large airway obstruction, or a persistent air leak. In these cases, an indwelling catheter might ensure symptom control.

3. *Ambulatory indwelling catheter*—available from different brands (e.g. PleurX, Rocket); patients or carers can be trained to connect either the brand-specific vacuum draining bottles or brand-specific adapters plus generic sterile urine collection bags at regular intervals (every few days to weekly). Alternatively

this can be performed by district nurses. The method has been shown to reduce length of hospitalization, allowing patients to stay in their own home or a nursing home.

The side effects include cellulitis, empyema, blockage, displacement, loculations, pneumothorax, and, rarely, tumour seeding of the catheter tract. In clinical practice the catheters are usually well tolerated. A spontaneous pleurodesis, possibly due to the foreign material, is reported in around half of all patients, which then allows the removal of the catheter.

The cost of the branded vacuum bottles is significant, and higher than the cost of adapter plus bag. Follow local guidelines regarding brands and draining option to be used. The costs are balanced by the avoidance of hospital admissions and improvement in the patient's quality of life. After insertion of an indwelling catheter, the patient should be discharged from hospital with a written information leaflet, clear instructions for patient, family and district nurses, and a supply of bottles or adapters plus drainage bags.

7. Is there any other recommendation post thoracoscopy, specifically for patients with mesothelioma?

Depending on the overall prognosis, prophylactic radiotherapy to the thoracoscopy/chest drain insertion site should be considered to reduce the risk of seeding and local recurrence, which otherwise is about 40%. According to the guideline there is little evidence to support this for pleural aspirations or pleural biopsy.

Further reading

Gasper WJ, Jamshidi R, Theodore PR. Palliation of thoracic malignancies. Surg Oncol. 2007 Dec;**16**(4):259–65.

Putnam JBJr, Walsh GL, Swisher SG, Roth JA, Suell DM, Vaporciyan AA, Smythe WR, Merriman KW, DeFord LL. Outpatient management of malignant pleural effusion by a chronic indwelling pleural catheter. Ann Thorac Surg. 2000 Feb;**69**(2):369–75.

Roberts ME, Neville E, Berrisford RG, Antunes G, Ali NJ; BTS Pleural Disease Guideline Group. Management of a malignant pleural effusion: British Thoracic Society pleural disease guideline 2010. Thorax. 2010 Aug;**65**(Suppl 2):ii32–40.

Index

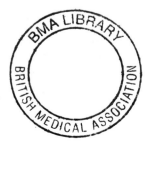